MOURAD BOUKHELOUA
SOUAD CHELGHOUM
OURIDA GACEM

SGLT2 INHIBITORS: EFFECTS ON CARDIOPROTECTION

MOURAD BOUKHELOUA
SOUAD CHELGHOUM
OURIDA GACEM

SGLT2 INHIBITORS: EFFECTS ON CARDIOPROTECTION

AND NEPHROPROTECTION

ScienciaScripts

Imprint
Any brand names and product names mentioned in this book are subject to trademark, brand or patent protection and are trademarks or registered trademarks of their respective holders. The use of brand names, product names, common names, trade names, product descriptions etc. even without a particular marking in this work is in no way to be construed to mean that such names may be regarded as unrestricted in respect of trademark and brand protection legislation and could thus be used by anyone.

Cover image: www.ingimage.com

This book is a translation from the original published under ISBN 978-620-6-70215-3.

Publisher:
Sciencia Scripts
is a trademark of
Dodo Books Indian Ocean Ltd. and OmniScriptum S.R.L publishing group

120 High Road, East Finchley, London, N2 9ED, United Kingdom
Str. Armeneasca 28/1, office 1, Chisinau MD-2012, Republic of Moldova, Europe
Printed at: see last page
ISBN: 978-620-7-14332-0

SGLT2 INHIBITORS:

EFFECTS IN CARDIOPROTECTION AND NEPHROPROTECTION

Pr MOURAD BOUKHELOUA

Pr SOUAD CHELGHOUM

Prof. OURIDA GACEM

FOREWORD

It is estimated that diabetes mellitus affects one in eleven adults worldwide. Despite the availability of many effective medications, only half of diabetic patients reach their individual HbA_{1c} target. There are many reasons for this, not least the lack of compliance observed in many patients. The wide range of therapeutic options and combinations available also makes medication management a complex task.

Sodium-glucose co-transporter type 2 (SGLT2) inhibitors are a new class of drugs currently used to treat patients with type 2 diabetes mellitus and heart failure. They have been shown to reduce the risk of worsening heart failure and improve the cardiovascular prognosis of diabetic patients at cardiovascular risk and those with renal failure.

The aim of this book is, on the one hand, to provide an overview of the studies on ISGLT2 with cardiovascular and renal endpoints conducted to date. To date, all studies have mainly assessed the safety of these antidiabetic agents in patients with established cardiovascular disease, with or without chronic renal insufficiency. Cardiovascular benefits, reduced mortality and improved renal function have all been clearly demonstrated.

CONTENTS

I. Introduction

Diabetes mellitus (DM) is a global health scourge that has reached alarming levels worldwide. Global diabetes prevalence was estimated at 9.3% (463 million people) in 2019 and is expected to reach 10.2% (578 million) by 2030 and 10.9% (700 million) by 2045 (1)Diabetes is one of the world's top 10 causes of death. Type 2 diabetes mellitus (T2DM) is the most common age-related metabolic disorder, affecting around 25% of people over 65 worldwide (2). The prevalence of T2DM has increased dramatically in recent decades and is considered one of the world's major health challenges (3). A metabolic syndrome may develop in type 2 diabetics through manifestations of overweight, obesity, hypertension and dyslipidemia (4). These metabolic abnormalities accompanying T2DM are associated with a high prevalence of chronic kidney disease (CKD), cardiovascular disease (CVD) and heart failure (HF), leading to high mortality and increased healthcare costs (4) (5).

T2DM mainly involves abnormal hepatic glucose metabolism, insulin resistance and increased glucose reabsorption by the kidneys, among others, leading to hyperglycemia (6). Chronic hyperglycemia leads to an increase in circulating free fatty acids and their uptake by myocardial cells; it also results in decreased glucose oxidation and increased myocardial oxygen consumption (7). This surplus of free fatty acids entering the myocardium causes deposition (lipotoxicity) and impaired mitochondrial ATP (adenosine triphosphate) synthesis (7). This can lead to diabetic cardiomyopathy, a condition that generally occurs in patients without hypertension or other risk factors for CI. It affects around 1.1% of diabetic patients, and is associated with a high mortality rate (8). Diabetic cardiomyopathy begins with left ventricular hypertrophy, followed by myocardial remodeling and abnormal filling of the left ventricle until the onset of PFEMI. If left untreated, the disease can progress to ICFER, characterized by decreased ventricular filling, reduced ventricular ejection fraction and increased ventricular wall stiffness (9).

Traditional anti-diabetic drugs that enhance or directly replace the action of insulin can lower blood glucose levels by facilitating the entry of glucose into cells, where it is then converted into glycogen, fat and protein (10) (11).

Recent advances in the understanding of diabetes have led to the development of sodium-glucose cotransporter 2 (SGLT2) inhibitors (ISGLT2). ISGLT2s have been shown to lower blood glucose levels by partially preventing the kidneys from reabsorbing glucose into the blood. They increase urinary glucose excretion, thereby improving diabetes control (12) (13). According to recent guidelines from the American Diabetes Association (ADA) and the American Association of Clinical Endocrinologists (AACE), these drugs play an important role, particularly in the treatment of T2DM with atherosclerotic cardiovascular disease (ASCVD), heart failure or chronic kidney disease (14) (15). In numerous large-scale clinical trials, these molecules have been shown to have remarkable effects on improving cardio-renal outcome in patients with or without T2DM, and in patients suffering from CHF with preserved or reduced ejection fraction (16) (17).

A number of mechanistic hypotheses have been proposed to explain the benefits of ISGLT2, such as the tubular hypothesis (18)the sodium hypothesis (19) and the "sparing substrate" hypothesis(20). More recently, the mechanism by which ISGLT2 protects organs has been proposed as a "water-sparing" response similar to that elicited by summer heat, enabling physiological adaptation to energy and water deprivation, thus prolonging the lifespan of vital organs (21). It is becoming increasingly clear that the mechanism underlying the cardio-renal benefits of ISGLT2 cannot be attributed to glycemic control alone.

Metabolic reprogramming, referring to the phenomenon in which cancer cells undergo metabolic adaptation to adverse environmental changes in order to meet the demands of survival and proliferation, has been described as one of the hallmarks of cancer (22). However, new evidence suggests that metabolic reprogramming is also involved in cardiovascular and renal diseases, which may contribute to disease progression and affect patient outcome (23) (24) (25).

In particular, ISGLT2 has been reported to induce a "fasting"-type metabolic pattern involving metabolic conversion from carbohydrates to other energy substrates and modulation of nutrient-sensing pathways, which may partly explain the cardio-renal protective effect of ISGLT2.

In this book, we will review normal cardiac and renal energy metabolism and the metabolic reprogramming involved in heart failure and diabetic nephropathy (DN). We will focus on the beneficial effects of SGLT2 inhibitors on metabolic reprogramming in cardio-renal disease, including the induction of a fasting-type metabolic paradigm and a transcriptional nutrient deprivation paradigm. We have combined recent advances from clinical trials and experimental studies and linked the cardio-renal protective effects of ISGLT2 to metabolic reprogramming and nutrient sensing offering, hopefully, broader insights and perspectives for future studies of these promising drugs.

II. Mechanisms of action of SGLT2 inhibitors

SGLTs belong to the mammalian solute carrier family 5 (SLC5), which comprises 12 members expressed in different tissues, responsible for the active transport of sugars, anions, vitamins and short-chain fatty acids (26). SGLT2 is a high-capacity, low-affinity cotransporter located in the S1 and S2 segments of the proximal tubule, responsible for the reabsorption of >90% of filtered glucose. SGLT1, on the other hand, is a low-capacity, high-affinity glucose transporter located in segment S3, which contributes to the reabsorption of the remaining glucose. Glucose reabsorption by SGLTs on the apical membrane of the proximal tubule is a secondary active transport process that depends on the driving force generated by the basolateral Na+/K+ -ATPase pump. Glucose is then transported via GLUT glucose transporters on the basolateral membrane into the bloodstream (27).

SGLT2 inhibitors significantly inhibit glucose and sodium reabsorption in the proximal tubule, resulting in increased urinary glucose excretion (with a low risk of hypoglycemia, unless combined with insulin, sulfonamide or glinide) and a slight osmotic diuresis, which is of interest since it causes contraction of both intravascular and interstitial fluid volume, unlike thiazide or loop diuretics, which act primarily on intravascular volume, which would explain its favorable cardiovascular effects in heart failure with reduced ejection fraction (ICFER), including in euvolemic patients at risk of developing acute functional renal failure under standard diuretic treatment (28). The potential mechanisms underlying the cardio-renal benefits of SGLT2 inhibitors are multiple, involving :

- Induction of diuresis/natriuresis, reduction of blood pressure to within 3 to 4 mm Hg of systolic value through natriuresis and direct arterial vasodilator effect, and improvement of cardiac load, which may occur in part through inhibition of sodium-hydrogen exchanger 3 and sympathetic tone (29,30);

- Reducing proximal sodium and glucose reabsorption, normalizing tubulo-glomerular *feedback* and lowering hyperfiltration (31) ;
- Mimicking systemic hypoxia and stimulating erythropoiesis, which can improve tissue oxygenation (32) ;
- Inhibition of SGLT1 (33);
- Anti-inflammation, reducing oxidative stress and apoptosis, and increasing autophagy due to a negative caloric balance induced by glycosuria, leading to a reduction in visceral and subcutaneous adipose tissue, which in turn reduces systemic inflammation and the production of pro-inflammatory cytokines (34,35) ;
- Improved cardiac energy metabolism through increased synthesis of ketone bodies, whose bioenergetic power is clearly superior to glucose and fatty acids, with reduced pathological remodeling (36);
- Increased circulating pro-angiogenic progenitor cells, which may contribute to improved vascular health (33) ;
- Lower cytoplasmic calcium and sodium levels, leading to improved contractility with reduced myocardial fibrosis and cardiac arrhythmia mortality (37).

The cardio-renal effects of SGLT2 inhibitors in major trials are summarized in Table 1.

III. Clinical evidence of the effect of SGLT2 inhibitors on metabolism and cardio-renal protection

More than two-thirds of people with T2D suffer from high blood pressure (hypertension). The coexistence of hypertension and T2DM significantly increases the risk of microvascular complications and cardiovascular consequences (38). Although lifestyle modifications, as well as antihypertensive treatment, are essential to reduce cardiovascular risk (38)some anti-hyperglycemic drugs may offer additional benefits in achieving blood pressure targets.

High levels of LDL cholesterol significantly increase the risk of atherosclerotic cardiovascular disease in patients with T2DM. Although the cornerstone of risk reduction is the use of statins, some anti-hyperglycemic drugs can also help reduce *lipoprotein* density *(LDL)* cholesterol (39). Various meta-analyses have shown that treatment with SGLT2 inhibitors reduces LDL cholesterol by around 0.2 to 2.3 mg/dl (40) (41).

Chronic hyperuricemia has been reported as an independent risk factor for diabetic CKD and cardiovascular disease (42). This is consistent with previous studies showing uric acid reductions of up to 0.9 mg/dl with dapagliflozin (43) (44).

Known for their pleiotropic effects, iSGLT2 is said to have a hypo-uricemic effect, with cardio-metabolic and renal benefits by reducing inflammation, as demonstrated by a study carried out in Canada involving T2DM and gout patients aged at least 18 years treated for one year or more with gliptin (n = 6,749) or iSGLT2 (n = 8,318). Over a mean follow-up of 1.6 years, the iSGLT2 group showed a 34% reduction in the recurrence rate of gout attacks compared with the iDDP4 group, with a 31% reduction in MI and a 48% reduction in hospitalizations or emergency room visits. Pathophysiologically, the hypo-uricemic effect is explained by glycosuria, which competes in the proximal tubule with GLUT 9-

mediated urate reabsorption, increasing uraturia. On the other hand, the intrinsic anti-inflammatory effect of hypo-uricemia is linked to the inhibition of interleukin 1β and the increase in SIRT-1, which confers a reduction in oxidative stress (45).

iSGLT2 has also shown promise in reducing the risk of atrial fibrillation (AF). However, the results are controversial and the underlying metabolic mechanism remains unclear. Emerging evidence suggests that iSGLT2 has additional beneficial metabolic effects on circulating metabolites beyond glycemic control, which may play a role in reducing AF risk. Several cohort studies have shown that total lipoprotein particle concentration and HDL particle concentration are associated with AF (46,47). Oxidative stress and chronic inflammation have been proposed as mediators of the protective effect of SGLT2 inhibition on AF, whereas previous data have suggested that HDL possesses anti-inflammatory and antioxidant properties (48-50). Furthermore, low HDL levels are an important component of the metabolic syndrome, which is associated with an increased risk of AF (47,51). Therefore, HDL could mediate this protective effect, but further studies are needed to better characterize this association.

A network meta-analysis of 38 clinical trials showed that, compared with placebo, in adults with type 2 diabetes, SGLT2 inhibitors can reduce glycated hemoglobin levels by 0.6 to 0.9%, fasting blood glucose levels by 1.1 to 1.9 mmol/L, body weight by 1.6 to 2.5 kg, systolic blood pressure by 2.8 to 4.9 mm Hg, diastolic blood pressure by 1.5 to 2.0 mm Hg, and raise high-density lipoprotein (HDL) cholesterol levels slightly by 0.05 to 0.07 mmol/L(52).

In terms of improving cardiovascular prognosis, a meta-analysis including three large cardiovascular prognosis trials and 34,322 T2DM patients showed that SGLT2 inhibitors reduced the risk of major adverse cardiovascular events by 11%, in MCVAS alone. SGLT2 inhibitors significantly reduced the risk of cardiovascular death or hospitalization for CI by 23%, with a similar benefit for patients with or without MCVAS (53). Even in patients without T2DM, SGLT2 inhibitors have been reported to significantly reduce the combined risk of CI exacerbation or cardiovascular death in patients with ICFER (17) (54).

Clinical Trials	**EMPA-REG OUTCOME**	**CANVAS Program**	**DECLARATION TIMI 58**	**VERTIS CV**	**DAPA HF**	**EMPEROR Reduced**	**SOLOIST WHE**	**EMPEROR Preserved**	**SCORED**	**CREDENCE**	**DAPA CKD**
Intervention	Empagifiozin	Canagliflozin	Dapagliflozin	Ertugliflozin	Dapagliflozin	Empagliflozin	Sotagliflozin	Empagliflozin	Sotagliflozin	Canagliflozin	Dapagliflozin
	10 or 25 mg vs placebo	300 or 100 mg vs placebo	10 mg vs placebo	5 or 15 mg vs placebo	10 mg vs placebo	10 mg vs placebo	200-400mg vs placebo	10 mg vs placebo	200-400mg vs placebo	100 mg vs placebo	10mg vs placebo
Population in)	7020	10,142	17,160	8246	4744	3730	1222	5988	10,584	4401	4304
Follow up (year)	3-1	3-6	4-2	3-5	2	0-7	0-75	2-18	1-33	2-6	2-4
T2DM (%)	100	100	100	100	42	49-8	100	49	100	100	67-5
ASCVD* or HEVEF	>99% with ASCVD	72-7% with ASCVD	40-6% with ASCVD	100% with ASCVD	100% with HFrEF	100% with HFrFF	100% with recent worsening HF	100% with HFpEF	19-9% with HFrEF	50-4% with ASCVD	37-4% with ASCVD
eGFR ml per min per 1 73m2)	>= 30	>= 30	>= 60	>= 30	>= 30	>= 20	>= 30	>= 20	25-60	30-89	25-75

Primary outcome (HR. 95%CI)	MACE 0-86 0-74--0-99	MACE 0 86 (0-75--0-97)	MACE 0 93 (0-84--1-03)	MACE 0.9 (0-85--1-11)	Worsening HF or cardiovascular death 0-74 (0-65--0-85)	Cardiovascular death or hospitalization for worsening HF:0-75 (0-65--0-86)	The total number of cardiovascular deaths and hospitalizations and urgent visits for HF:0-67 (0-52--0-85)	A composite of cardiovascular death or hospitalization for HF:0-79 0.09--0-90)	The total number of cardiovascular deaths and hospitalizations and urgent visits for HF:0-74 (0-63--0-88)	ESRD. doubling of the Sc level or renal or cardiovascular death 70 0-59--0-82	A sustained decline in the eGFR _50% ESRD, or renal or cardiovascular death 0.61 (0.51--0-72)
Cardiovascular death (HR. 95%CI)	0-62 (0-49--0-77)	0-87 (072--1-06)	0-98 (0-82--1-17)	0-92 (0-77--1-11)	0-82 (0-69--0-98)	0-92 (0-75--1-12)	0-84 (0-58--1-22)	0-91 (0-76--1-09)	0-90 (0-73--1-12)	0-78 (0-61--1-00)	0-81 (0-58--1-12)
All-cause mortality (HR, 95%CI)	0-68 (0-57--0-82)	0-87 (0-74--1-01)	0-93 (0-82--1-04)	0-93 (0-80--1-08)	0-83 (0-71--0-97)	0-92 (0-77--1-10)	0-82 (0-59--1-14)	1-00 (0-87--1-15)	0-99 (0-83--1-18)	0-83 (0-68--1-02)	0-69 (0-53--0-88)
Hospitalization for HF (HR 95%CI)	0-65 (0-50--0-85)	0-67 (0-52--0-87)	0-73 (0-61-0-88)	0-70 (0-54--0-90)	0-70 (0-59--0-83)	0-69 (0-59-0-81)	/	0-71 (0-60--0-83)	0-67 (0-55--0-82)	0-61 (0-47--0-80)	/
Renal outcomes (HR, 95%CD)	/	Progression of albuminuria: 0-73 (0-67--0-79); Sustained 40% discount	>= 40% decrease in eGFR to 60 mL per min per 1-73m 2 ESRD or renal death	Death from renal causes RRT. doubling of the Sc level 0-81 (0-63--1-04)	A sustained decline in the eGFR >=50 % or ESRD or renal Death : 0 -71 (0-44--1-16)	Mean slope of change in eGFR per year -0-55 vs. -2-28 mL per min per 1.73m 2(P<0 01)	Mean change in eGFR - 0-16 (-1-30--0-98)	Mean slope of change in eGFR year: -1-25 vs -2-62m per min 1.73 m2 (P<0-01)	A sustained decline in the eGFR >=50 % from baseline gold sustained eGFR< 15 mL per min	ESRD, doubling of the Scr level or renal death : 0-66(0-53--0-81)	Decline in eGFR >=50 % ESRD, or renal death : 0-56 (0-45--0-68)

		in eGFR RRT, or renal death 0-60 (0-47--0-77)	0-53 (0-43--0-66)						per 1.73m 2 for >= 30 days RRT		

Table 1: Large-scale clinical trials of SGLT2 inhibitors on the incidence of adverse cardio-renal events. ASCVD*: atherosclerotic cardiovascular disease, involving the coronary, cerebrovascular or peripheral arterial systems; HFrEFy: heart failure with reduced ejection fraction (New York Heart Association class IIIV and an LVEF of 40%); HFpEFz: heart failure with preserved ejection fraction (New York Heart Association class IIIV and an LVEF of 40%). HFpEFz: heart failure with preserved ejection fraction (New York Heart Association class IIIV and LVEF>40%); MACEx: major adverse cardiovascular events, representing a composite of death from cardiovascular causes, non-fatal myocardial infarction or non-fatal stroke. Abbreviations: EMPA-REG OUTCOME: Empagliflozin Cardiovascular Outcome Event Trial in T2DM Patients; CANVAS Program: Canagliflozin Cardiovascular Assessment Study Program; DECLARE-TIMI 58: Dapagliflozin Effect on Cardiovascular Events-Thrombosis in Myocardial Infarction 58; VERTIS CV: Evaluation of Ertugliflozin Efficacy and Safety Cardiovascular Outcomes Trial; DAPA-HF: Dapagliflozin and Prevention of Adverse Outcomes in Heart Failure Trial; EMPEROR-Reduced: Empagliflozin Outcome Trial in Patients with Chronic Heart Failure with Reduced Ejection Fraction; SOLOIST-WHF: The Effect of Sotagliflozin on Cardiovascular Events in Patients with Type 2 Diabetes Post Worsening Heart Failure Trial; EMPEROR-PRESERVED: Empagliflozin Outcome Trial in Patients with Chronic Heart Failure with Preserved Ejection Fraction; SOLOIST-WHF: The Effect of Sotagliflozin on Cardiovascular Events in Patients with Type 2 Diabetes Post Worsening Heart Failure Trial Heart Failure with Preserved Ejection Fraction; EMPEROR-PRESERVED. Empagliflozin Outcome Trial in Patients with Chronic Heart Failure with Preserved Ejection Fraction SCORED: Trial of the Effect of Sotagliflozin on Cardiovascular and Renal Events in Patients with Type 2 Diabetes and Moderate Renal Failure at Cardiovascular Risk; CREDENCE: Canagliflozin and Renal Events in Diabetes and Established Nephropathy Clinical Evaluation Trial; DAPA-CKD: Dapagliflozin and Prevention of Adverse Outcomes in Chronic Kidney Disease Trial; SGLT2: sodium-glucose co-transporter 2; T2DM: type 2 diabetes mellitus; HF: heart failure; eGFR: estimated glomerular filtration rate; HR: hazard ration; CI: confidence interval; RRT: renal-replacement therapy; ESRD: end-stage renal disease; CKD: chronic kidney disease; Scr: serum creatinine.

More encouragingly, in T2DM patients with recent exacerbations of heart failure, it was also found that initiation of SGLT2 inhibitors immediately after the onset of heart failure significantly reduced overall cardiovascular mortality and hospitalization for heart failure (55) (56).

The DAPA HF and EMPEROR trials investigated the impact of SGLT2 inhibitors in heart failure patients with or without diabetes. The DAP HF study randomized 4744 patients with NYHA class II to IV heart failure symptoms and a left ventricular ejection fraction <40% to treatment with dapaglifozine 10 mg daily or placebo. During 18.2 months of follow-up, the primary endpoint (worsening heart failure - either hospitalization for heart failure or urgent visit when the patient required intravenous treatment for heart failure) or CV death was reduced by 26% (HR 0.74 95% CI 0.65-0.85). Worsening heart failure was reduced by 30% and CV death by 18% (HR 0.82 95% CI 0.69-0.98). Similar benefits were observed in more than 50% of non-diabetic patients and diabetic patients with or without

ischemic cause of heart failure. An improvement in functional status was reported in patients receiving dapaglifozine. There was no increase in the incidence of volume depletion, renal dysfunction or hypoglycemia in the dapaglifozine-treated group compared with the placebo-treated group. (57).

The EMPEROR Reduced trial included 3,730 patients with NYHA class II-IV heart failure symptoms and an ejection fraction of less than 40%, who were randomized to receive either empagliflozin or placebo. Patients receiving empagliflozin and followed for a median of 16 months showed a 25% reduction in the primary endpoint of hospitalization for heart failure or cardiovascular death (HR 0.75 95% CI0.65-0.86). Hospitalization for heart failure was reduced by 30%, but CV mortality was not significantly reduced (HR 0.92 95% CI 0.75-1.12). Similar reductions in the primary endpoint were observed in diabetic and non-diabetic patients. The decline in eGFR was slower in patients treated with empagliflozin (58).

A recent outcome trial of empagliflozin in patients with chronic heart failure with preserved ejection fraction (HFpEF) (EMPEROR-PRESERVED) showed that empagliflozin reduced the combined risk of cardiovascular death or hospitalization for CHF in patients with HFpEF, irrespective of the presence or absence of diabetes (59). Another randomized controlled trial (RCT), the DELIVER trial (Dapagliflozin Evaluation to Improve the Lives of Patients with Preserved Ejection Fraction Heart Failure, NCT03619213), is currently underway to confirm the cardiovascular benefit of SGLT2 inhibitors in patients with ICFEP (60).

In renal outcome trials, SGLT2 inhibitors have been shown to reduce the relative risk of renal damage in patients with T2DM. Prevention of adverse outcomes in chronic kidney disease (DAPA-CKD) was discontinued early due to its apparent "overwhelming effect" on reducing the risk of renal complications with or without T2DM (61).

Dapagliflozin significantly reduces the urinary albumin/creatinine ratio and improves estimated glomerular filtration rate (eGFR). This lasting benefit has been demonstrated in clinical trials and meta-analyses (43,44) (62). In addition, the DECLARE-TIMI 58 trial showed that dapagliflozin had a beneficial effect on renal events, resulting in a significant 24% reduction in events on the composite endpoint which includes a reduction > 40% in eGFR to < 60 ml/min /1.73 m^2, the occurrence of new end-stage renal failure or death from renal or cardiovascular causes (63). This positive effect was also observed in CKD patients (DAPA CKD trial), irrespective of the presence of diabetes (61).

EMPA-KIDNEY (Cardiac and Renal Protection Study of Empagliflozin, NCT03594110) is underway to test whether empagliflozin can improve cardio-renal outcome in a larger number of CKD patients, particularly those with overt albuminuria and eGFR <20 ml/1.73 m^2/minute (64).

- In parallel, another promising molecule, "AR-GLP1", which offers better glycemic control by improving β-cell function by promoting their proliferation and inhibiting their apoptosis, has also proved interesting for its cardio and nephroprotective effects, as revealed by Anson et al. Using a retrospective cohort on an international database (TriNetX) encompassing almost 125 million patients, of whom 26,311 (13%) of the 196,691 T1DM included were put on non-insulin treatments (metformin, AR-GLP1 and iSGLT2), the researchers then focused on patients who had been taking AR-GLP1 or iSGLT2 for six months or more, with a total of 933 in each arm; the results five years later were encouraging, with a greater reduction in weight (-2.4 kg vs. +1.5 kg) and eGFR (+3.5 mL/min/1.73 m^2 vs. -7.2 mL/min/1.73 m^2), thereby reducing the risk of developing heart failure (RR 0,44 [CI95% 0.23-0.83], p = 0.0092) or chronic kidney disease (RR 0.49 [CI95% 0.28-0.86], p = 0.0118) by iSGL2 and HBA1c value (-0.5% vs -0.2%) by AR-GLP1 ; this major study highlighted the metabolic benefit of AR-GLP1 and the cardio-renal protection of iSGLT2 in type 1 diabetics, with a favorable benefit-risk ratio offering promising therapeutic options (reference).

IV. Energy metabolism in the normal heart and metabolic reprogramming in heart failure

1. Energy metabolism in the normal heart

The heart, described as a "metabolic omnivore", is capable of metabolizing fatty acids (FAs), carbohydrates (glucose and lactate), ketone bodies and amino acids according to supply, to ensure the replenishment of adenosine triphosphate (ATP) to meet contractile demand. In the adult heart, mitochondria occupy more than a third of the volume of the cardiomyocyte, and mitochondrial oxidative phosphorylation contributes more than 95% of ATP production, with glycolysis providing the remaining 5% (65). Under normoxic conditions, fatty acid oxidation (OAG) is the main energy source, providing around 40-60% of the ATP required to meet contractile demand, it is an energy source, providing around 40-60% of total ATP, followed by carbohydrate oxidation (20-40%), with only modest utilization (10-15%) of ketone bodies or branched-chain amino acids (BCAAs) (66).

GAs are transported into cardiomyocytes in part via GA translocase differentiation cluster 36 (CD36) and plasma membrane GA-binding protein (FABP), then esterified to fatty acyl-CoA by fatty acyl-CoA synthetase (FACS) (65). Over 80% of the fatty acyl-CoA is then transferred to the mitochondria with the aid of carnitine, and unused GAs are mainly stored as triglycerides.

Carnitine palmitoyl transferase 1 (CPT-1) is the rate-limiting enzyme in this process. Next, fatty acyl-CoA undergoes b-oxidation, generating acetyl-CoA, which enters the tricarboxylic acid (TCA) cycle and produces nicotinamide adenine dinucleotide (NADH) and flavin adenine dinucleotide (FADH2) for oxidative phosphorylation (OXPHOS) and ATP production (66).

Fatty acid oxidation is strongly regulated by various mechanisms, such as substrate availability, intermediary metabolites (e.g.

malonyl CoA can induce CPT-1 inhibition), post-translational modification of key enzymes and the regulation of

transcription of genes linked to this oxidation, helping to ensure the high energy demand for cardiac work (66).

Glucose is another important fuel for the heart, mainly taken up by the cardiomyocyte isotype 4 glucose transporter (GLUT4), followed by the cardiomyocyte isotype 1 glucose transporter (GLUT1).

After entering myocardial cells, glucose is phosphorylated by hexokinase to form glucose-6-phosphate (G-6-P) and then converted to pyruvate, producing ATP from cytoplasmic glycolysis and mitochondrial aerobic oxidation.

The pyruvate generated by glycolysis can be converted to lactate by the enzyme lactate dehydrogenase (LDH). Lactate can also be taken up by cardiomyocytes via the monocarboxylate transporter 1 (MCT1), which exports lactate, then converts it to pyruvate to enter the mitochondria via the mitochondrial pyruvate transporter (MPC), which serves as an energy substrate for the heart.

Ketone bodies are produced in the liver and used in extra-hepatic tissues. b-Hydroxybutyrate (b-OHB) is the predominant ketone body used in the heart, and is taken up by cardiomyocytes via SLC16A1.

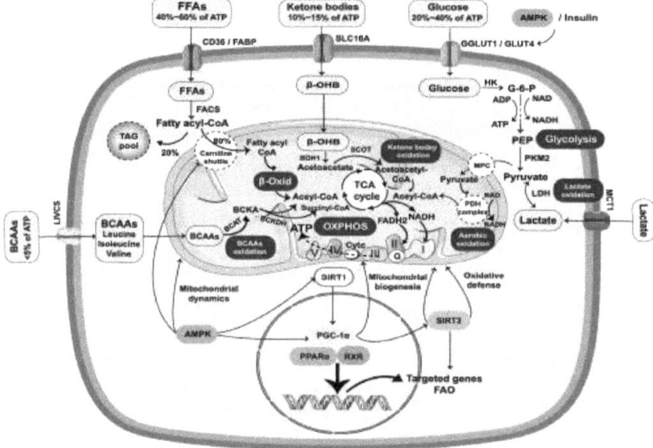

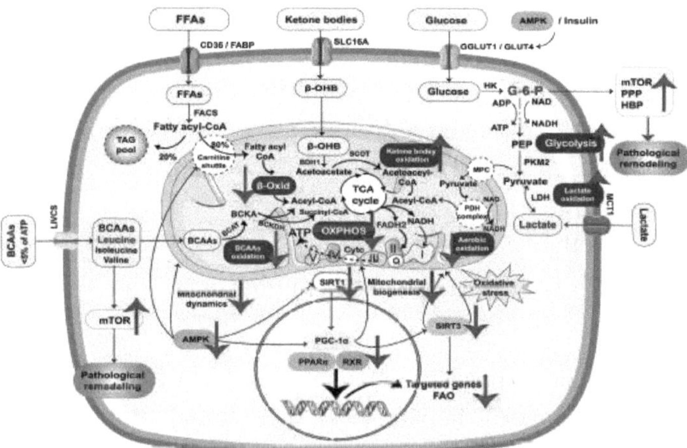

Figure 1: Energy metabolism in the normal heart and heart failure (a). In the normal heart, GAs are the main substrate for cardiac ATP production, while carbohydrates (glucose and lactate), ketone bodies and BCAAs play a lesser role (b). In CI, myocardial substrate utilization shifts from GAs to carbohydrates (particularly glycolysis). The uncoupling of glycolysis and glucose oxidation, and the reduced catabolism of cardiac BCAAs, lead to the accumulation of glycolytic intermediates and polycyclic fatty acids (BCAAs) (leucine). BCAA (leucine), activating the mTOR signalling pathway, which contributes to insulin resistance and pathological remodelling. In addition, the myocardium increasingly relies on ketone bodies as an alternative fuel. Nutrient deprivation sensors, including SIRT1 and AMPK, are suppressed in heart failure, leading to reduced FAO, altered mitochondrial biogenesis and dynamics, and

increased oxidative stress via effects on insulin resistance. Increased oxidative stress through effects on downstream transcriptional regulators (mainly PCG-1a). Abbreviations: FFA:fatty acid free; ATP: adenosine triphosphate; ADP: adenosine diphosphate; CD36: differentiation cluster 36; FABP: fatty acid binding protein; CoA: coenzyme A; FACS: fatty acyl-CoA synthetase; TAG: triglyceride; b-Oxid: b-oxidation; b-OHB: b-hydroxybutyrate; BDH1: b-hydroxybutyrate dehydrogenase-1; SCOT: succinyl-CoA: 3-oxoacid CoA transferase; TCA: tricarboxylic acid; AMPK: adenosine monophosphate-activated protein kinase; GLUT1: glucose transporter 1; GLUT4: glucose transporter 4; HK: hexokinase; G-6-P: glucose-6-phosphate; PEP: phosphoenolpyruvate; PKM2: pyruvate kinase; LDH: lactate dehydrogenase; MCT1: monocarboxylic acid transporter 1; MPC: mitochondrial pyruvate carrier; PDH: pyruvate dehydrogenase; FADH2: flavin adenine dinucleotide; NADH: nicotinamide adenine dinucleotide; OXPHOS: oxidative phosphorylation; Q: coenzyme Q; Cytc: cytochrome c; BCAA: branched-chain amino acid; LIVCS: branched-chain amino acid:cation symporter; BCAT: branched-chain amino acid aminotransferase; BCKA: branched-chain ketoacid; BCKDH: branched-chain alpha-ketoacid dehydrogenase; SIRT1: silent information regulator 1; PGC-1a: PPARa: peroxisome proliferator-activated receptor-gamma co-activator 1a; RXR: retinoid X receptors; FAO: fatty acid oxidation; SIRT3: silent information regulator 3; mTOR: mechanistic target of rapamycin; PPP: pentose phosphate pathway; HBP: hexosamine biosynthetic pathway.

The b-OHB is then converted to acetoacetate by b-hydroxybutyrate dehydrogenase 1 (BDH1) and activated by succinyl-CoA:3-oxoacid CoA transferase (SCOT) to form acetoacetyl CoA; the latter undergoes a thiolysis process to form acetyl-CoA and then enters the TCA cycle to produce the ATP required for cardiac contraction (67).

AACRs (leucine, valine and isoleucine) are also readily used as fuel in cells other than hepatocytes. The initial step in AACR metabolism is transamination to form branched-chain a-keto acids (CACRs) via branched-chain aminotransferases (ATCRs). CACRs then undergo irreversible oxidative decarboxylation via branched-chain a-keto acid dehydrogenase (CCRDH) complexes to form acetyl-CoA or succinyl-CoA, which then enter the Krebs cycle to produce ATP (68). The energy metabolism of the normal heart is illustrated in Figure 1a.

2. Metabolic reprogramming in heart failure

In heart failure (HF), energy metabolism is disrupted, and metabolic flexibility is impaired, along with altered mitochondrial function and oxidative metabolism, leading to a state of "energy deprivation" (66,67).

The myocardial energy substrate shifts from GAs to carbohydrates (particularly glycolysis) to adapt to the reduced oxygen and energy demand, consistent with the reinduction of a fetal-type metabolic mode (69).

The increase in glycolysis is consistent with the increase in GLUT1 expression to accelerate glucose uptake, but is insufficient to compensate for the energy deficit. Furthermore, the uncoupling of glycolysis from glucose oxidation leads to the accumulation of glycolytic intermediates. Among these, G-6-P, recently found to be controlled by phosphoglucose isomerase activity, could serve as an activator of the mechanistic target of rapamycin (mTOR) complex 1 (mTORC1) and also fuel accessory pathways, such as the hexosamine biosynthetic pathway and the pentose phosphate pathway, thus exacerbating pathological myocardial remodeling (70).

In addition, recent studies indicate that the myocardium is increasingly dependent on ketone bodies as an alternative fuel in advanced heart failure (71).

Murashige et al. (72) found that ICFER patients had almost tripled their ketone body consumption (16.4% vs. 6.4%), and doubled lactate consumption (5.0% vs. 2.8%), with a reduction in fatty acid oxidation from 85.9% to 71.4%.

Given that the phosphorus/oxygen ratio of ketones (2.50) is higher than that of palmitate (2.33), this change in substrate preference may represent an adaptive mechanism in ICFER. In contrast to ICFER, a recent study developed a mouse model of ICFEP and found a reduction in b-OHB oxidation, indicating that the use of ketone bodies may not contribute to its benefits in ICFEP.

Interestingly, they found that mitochondrial hyperacetylation and inflammation are key factors in the pathogenesis of ICFEP, which could be ameliorated by increasing the level of b-OHB (73)Future studies are needed to explore the exact role of ketone bodies in ICFEP and their potential mechanisms.

In addition, elevated levels of circulating and cardiac AACR have also been observed in CI, as well as a decrease in cardiac catabolism of AACR (74). Using coronary artery ligation, inducing myocardial infarction (MI) in mouse models, Wang et al. (75) found that impaired cardiac catabolism of AACRs directly contributed to post-MI cardiac dysfunction and remodeling, which may be partly due to activation of mTOR signaling. Furthermore, enhancement of AACR catabolism using BT2 (3,6-dichlorobenzo[b]thiophene-2-carboxylic acid), a CCRDH kinase inhibitor, improved cardiac systolic contractility and diastolic mechanics in a murine model of heart failure, indicating that targeting AACR catabolism could be a novel and potentially effective treatment for heart failure (76).

In humans with established CI, altered AACR oxidation was also found to be associated with cardiac insulin resistance (77). How changes in AACR metabolism alter heart failure remains incompletely understood, and the importance of AACRs in the pathogenesis of heart failure requires further investigation.

Furthermore, in the failing heart, oxidative metabolism in mitochondria is impaired, leading to a state of intracellular nutrient surplus, which would suppress nutrient starvation sensors, including silent information regulator 1 (SIRT1) and adenosine monophosphate-activated protein kinase (AMPK). SIRT1, a nicotinamide adenine dinucleotide-dependent deacetylase, acts as a master switch controlling the gluconeogenesis/glycolysis relationship and lipid metabolism, as well as maintaining mitochondrial quality through its action on downstream substrates (78). Activation of AMPK increases the rate of catabolism and decreases the rate of anabolism to promote ATP production, in part by inhibiting mTORC1 (79). Peroxisome proliferator-activated receptor gamma co-activator 1a (PGC-1a), a master transcriptional regulator of lipid metabolism and mitochondrial function, could be activated by SIRT1 via deacetylation or AMPK via phosphorylation.

The effects of PGC-1a are manifold (80)such as (a) promotion of mitochondrial biogenesis and mitochondrial DNA replication, (b) optimization of mitochondrial dynamics, (c) defense against oxidative stress via activation of SIRT3, and (d) stimulation of GA oxidation via peroxisome proliferator-activated receptors (PPARs) and retinoid X receptors (RXRs).

Under CI conditions, PGC-1a expression is repressed, correlating with mitochondrial dysfunction, increased oxidative stress and reduced GA oxidation. Energy metabolism in CI is illustrated in figure 1b.

V. Renal energy metabolism and metabolic reprogramming in diabetic nephropathy

1. Energy metabolism in the normal kidney

The kidney is the most metabolically active organ after the heart, requiring large amounts of ATP to eliminate waste and reabsorb most of the filtered water and solutes (81). It is responsible for different metabolic programs in different parts of the nephron. The renal medulla mainly exhibits a high rate of glycolysis due to its low oxygen content and low amounts of oxidative enzymes, whereas the renal cortex, composed of a large number of proximal tubules, relies more heavily on OAG and gluconeogenesis (82).

More specifically, the proximal tubule is responsible for the reabsorption of approximately 70% of the fluids and solutes filtered by the glomerulus, and generates ATP primarily through the aerobic metabolism of various substrates, including GAs, glutamine, pyruvate, citrate and lactate (83). In contrast, distal tubules are totally dependent on anaerobic glycolysis to generate ATP (84) due to the low oxygen content of the renal medulla. The energy metabolism of renal tubular epithelial cells (RTECs) is illustrated in Figure 2a.

2. Metabolic reprogramming in diabetic nephropathy

Diabetic nephropathy (DN) is a chronic microvascular complication of diabetes and one of the main causes of end-stage renal disease (ESRD) (85). The pathophysiology of diabetic nephropathy is complex, multifactorial and heterogeneous. Alterations in the renal metabolic network caused by hyperglycemia and dyslipidemia play a crucial role. Sass et al.(86) using metabolic flux analysis, found that tricarboxylic acid cycle (TCA) and glycolytic flux were higher in the diabetic renal cortex of db/db mice than in control mice. Furthermore, increased metabolism in the early stages of ND was shown to be associated with dysfunction of the mitochondrial electron transport chain, leading to less efficient ATP production and progression of ND.

a. Energetic metabolism of TECs in the normal kidney

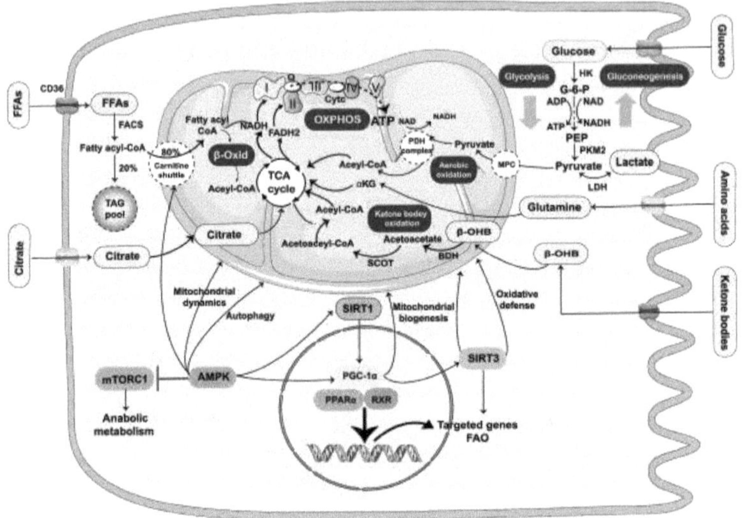

b. Energetic metabolic reprogramming of TECs in the diabetic kidney

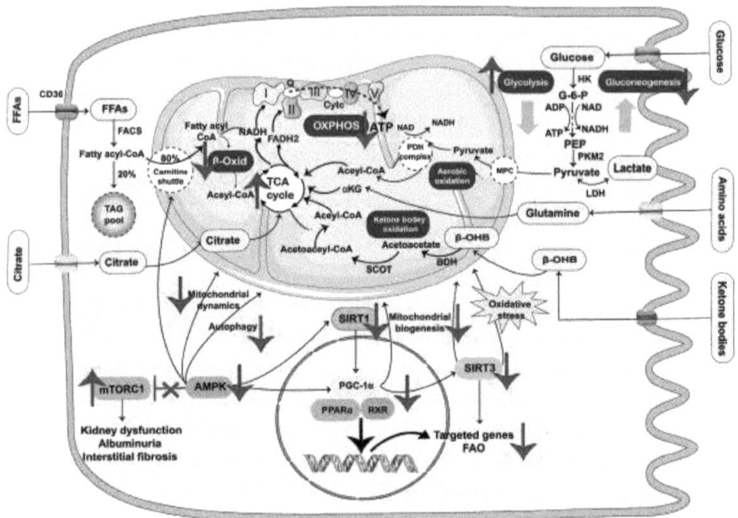

Figure 2: Energy metabolism in TECs from normal and diabetic kidneys.

(a). TECs generate ATP primarily through the aerobic metabolism of various substrates, including GAs, glutamine, pyruvate, citrate and lactate, which are metabolized to acetyl-CoA before entering the TCA cycle. Proximal TECs produce ATP mainly via

FAO, and also participate in the gluconeogenesis process. In contrast, distal tubules rely primarily on anaerobic glycolysis to generate ATP. (b). In DKD, the metabolic program switches from CAM to glycolysis. Levels of key CAM-related transcriptional regulators and enzymes were significantly down-regulated in proximal TECs. Lipid accumulation due to decreased FAO or increased FA synthesis contributes to the development of DKD. The mTOR and AMPK signaling pathways play an important role in the progression of DKD, involving the regulation of energy homeostasis and mitochondrial function. mTORC1 was found to be activated in proximal TECs of the diabetic kidney, leading to renal dysfunction, albuminuria and interstitial fibrosis. AMPK may participate in the regulation of mitochondrial biogenesis by stimulating the PGC-1a protein. In addition, AMPK stimulates catabolic metabolism and activates autophagy by inhibiting mTORC1 under conditions of nutrient deprivation. Abbreviations: TEC: tubular epithelial cell; ATP: adenosine triphosphate; CoA: coenzyme A; TCA: tricarboxylic acid; FAO: fatty acid oxidation; TCA: hydrochloric acid. tricarboxylic acid; FAO: fatty acid oxidation; FFA: free fatty acid; CD36: differentiation cluster 36; ADP: adenosine diphosphate; FACS: fatty acylCoA synthetase; TAG: triglyceride; b-Oxid: b-oxidation; HK: hexokinase; G-6-P: glucose-6-phosphate; PEP: phosphoenolpyruvate; PKM2: pyruvate kinase; LDH: lactate dehydrogenase; aKG: a-ketoglutarate; b-OHB: b-hydroxybutyrate; BDH1: b- hydroxybutyrate dehydrogenase-1; SCOT: succinyl-CoA: 3-oxoacid CoA transferase; MPC: mitochondrial pyruvate transporter; PDH: pyruvate dehydrogenase; FADH2: flavin adenine dinucleotide; NADH: nicotinamide adenine dinucleotide; OXPHOS: oxidative phosphorylation; Q: coenzyme Q; Cytc: cytochrome c; mTOR: mechanistic target of rapamycin; SIRT1: silent information regulator 1; PGC-1a : peroxisome proliferator-activator receptor PGC-1a: peroxisome proliferator-activated receptor-gamma co-activator 1a; PPARa: peroxisome proliferator-activated receptor a; RXR: retinoid X receptors; SIRT3: silent information regulator 3.

In terms of renal glucose reabsorption, the proximal convoluted tubule plays a central role in sodium-glucose bound transport, accounting for 60% of renal energy expenditure. In particular, proximal tubular epithelial cells (PTECs) consume almost two-thirds of reabsorbed energy (83). In the diabetic context, glucose reabsorption by CETPs is enhanced by hyperglycemia due to increased regulation of SGLT2 (87). In mice with ND, increased glucose reabsorption by CETPs leads to a state of hypernutrition, which activates nutrient-sensing pathways in these cells, resulting in renal dysfunction, proteinuria and interstitial fibrosis (88).

The current dogma is that the beneficial effects of SGLT2 inhibitors are primarily a hemodynamic effect on the nephron, mediated by glomerular feedback, leading to relative arteriolar vasoconstriction and hence lower glomerular filtration pressure (89). However, this hypothesis has not been verified in more recent human studies (90). The effects of ISGLT2, including reduced hypoxia, inflammation and serum uric acid toxicity, may play a role in the renoprotection of ISGLT2 (91). In conclusion, the exact molecular mechanism underlying the robust renal protective effect of ISGLT2 remains unclear.

CETPs rely on oxidative phosphorylation to generate the ATP required for glucose and sodium transport. In diabetes, hyperglycemia increases the sodium reabsorption workload of CETP, most likely through increased expression of SGLT2 in these cells (87)This increases glomerular filtration of glucose, followed by reabsorption by CETP (92) . We hypothesize that this leads to persistent activation of nutrient-sensing pathways in CETPs, which may contribute to the development and progression of ND.

The rapamycin-sensitive mTOR complex (mTORC1) integrates signals from nutrients, primarily glucose and branched-chain amino acids (BCAAs), to control protein synthesis, cell size, proliferation and autophagy (93). Here, we identify mTORC1 activation as one of the primary drivers of ND evolution, which promotes fibrogenesis formation. ISGLT2 treatment inhibits mTORC1 and prevents renal dysfunction. We also show that gene activation of mTORC1 in vivo mimics alterations in ND and neutralizes the protective effects of ISGLT2, while gene repression of mTORC1 mirrors the effects of ISGLT2 and protects against fibrogenesis and renal failure. Collectively, these results suggest that the RPTC mTORC1 plays a central role **in** the pathophysiology of ND and mediates the beneficial effects of ISGLT2.

In diabetic kidneys, the metabolic program shifts from OAG to glycolysis (86,94). In ND, Cai et al. (94) found a significantly high accumulation of lipids in the tubulointerstitial space of microdissected human kidney samples. Furthermore, ND patients had significantly lower levels of the transcriptional regulator, peroxisome proliferator Activated Receptors (PPARa) and the key OAG-associated enzyme, carnitine palmitoyl transferase 1 (CPT-1) than non-diabetic patients. Lipid accumulation due to decreased OAG or increased GA synthesis also contributes to nephropathy in metabolic diseases (95). The progression of ND to renal fibrosis has been reported to be characterized by a shift from OAG metabolism to glycolysis and lipid accumulation, which is associated with increased expression of Hipoxia Inducible Factor 1alfa (HIF-1a), leading to tubulointerstitial inflammation (94) (96).

In particular, two nutrient-sensing pathways in the kidney have been extensively studied: mechanistic target of rapamycin (mTOR) signaling and adenosine monophosphate-activated protein kinase (AMPK). These two signaling pathways play a role in the regulation of energy homeostasis and mitochondrial function (97,98). The mTORC1 pathway, activated by nutrient availability (mainly glucose and amino acids), has been shown to be activated in diabetic kidney CETP, leading to renal dysfunction, proteinuria and interstitial fibrosis (88). Moreover, mTORC1 overactivation has been shown to be closely associated with podocyte injury in ND through increased cytotoxicity and inhibition of autophagy, suggesting that inhibition of mTORC1 overactivation could be a promising therapeutic approach in proteinuric and non-proteinuric ND (99).

AMPK is involved in the regulation of mitochondrial biogenesis by stimulating peroxisome proliferator-activated receptor-gamma co-activator 1alfa (PGC-1a). Furthermore, AMPK stimulates catabolism and activates autophagy by inhibiting mTORC1 under nutrient-deficient conditions, providing another therapeutic target for metabolic dysfunction in ND (98). The metabolic **energetic** reprogramming of epithelial tubular cells (ETCs) in diabetic kidneys is illustrated in figure 2b.

VI. Cardio-renal protection of SGLT2 inhibitors based on metabolic reprogramming

1. SGLT2 inhibitors induce a fasting-type metabolic paradigm

Since SGLT2 is the most important mediator of filtered glucose reabsorption, selective inhibition of SGLT2 induces glycosuria and increases net urinary caloric loss by around 200-300 k cal per day, despite compensatory upregulation of SGLT1. Caloric loss mediated by SGLT2 inhibition mimics a fasting-type metabolic paradigm, which further elicits adaptive whole-body energy metabolism responses involving glucose homeostasis, hormone release, fuel selection and energy expenditure (100).

The direct metabolic effect of SGLT2 inhibitors has been shown to induce a decrease in blood glucose levels, leading to a decrease in insulin secretion and an increase in glucagon, as well as a paradoxical increase in endogenous glucose production (PEG) (101). The mechanisms underlying the increase in PEG are not yet known and may be attributed to (a) increased glucagon levels and the glucagon/insulin ratio (102)(b) direct inhibition of SGLT2 in pancreatic a-cells for glucagon secretion, (c) increased gluconeogenesis (103) and (d) a neural loop between kidney and liver to stimulate hepatic glucose production. Increased PEG can potentially counteract the hypoglycemic power of SGLT2 inhibitors, thereby reducing the risk of hypoglycemia.

In parallel with the reduction in insulin secretion, b-cell function and insulin sensitivity throughout the body and periphery were significantly improved, which may be partly due to the rapid reduction in glucotoxicity and the chronic reduction in body weight (101,104).

SGLT2 inhibitors were also found to exert indirect protective effects on the kidney and heart, independent of the direct effects of SGLT2 inhibition, at least in part. Metabolome analysis of diabetic mice showed that ipragliflozin reversed the accumulation of Krebs cycle intermediates and the increase in oxidative stress in the renal cortex, corresponding to the amelioration of glomerular damage. However, similar ipragliflozin-induced effects were not observed in the medulla interna, future studies are needed to clarify the differential metabolic effects of SGLT2 inhibitors in different regions of the kidney (105).

Furthermore, after chronic treatment with SGLT2 inhibitors, lipolysis, lipid oxidation and ketogenesis became more marked in both diabetic and non-diabetic patients, suggesting a progressive shift in fuel utilization from carbohydrates to GAs and ketone bodies (106).

High levels of GA are used for the hepatic formation of ketone bodies, which are energy-efficient substrates, and will be absorbed by the heart and kidneys, improving myocardial and renal epithelial performance (107). To date, the detailed molecular mechanisms by which SGLT2 inhibitors contribute to increased ketone body levels, and the mechanisms underlying elevated ketone body utilization in damaged kidneys and myocardium remain unclear. Further research is needed to answer these questions. The effects of SGLT2i on energy metabolism are shown in Figure 3.

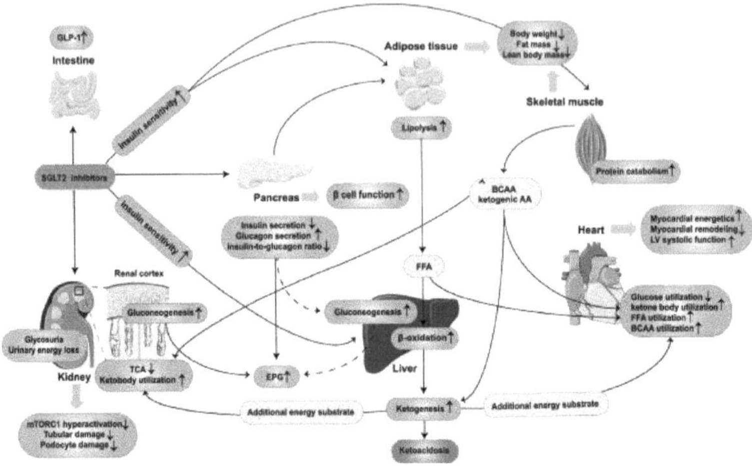

Fig. 3: Effects of SGLT2 inhibitors on energy metabolism. Treatment with SGLT2 inhibitors results in glycosuria and a net loss of urinary energy, as well as reduced insulin levels and increased glucagon and GLP-1 levels. Despite the reduction in insulin secretion, b-cell function and insulin sensitivity throughout the body and in peripheral tissues improved. Increased glucagon levels and a decreased insulin-glucagon ratio lead to an increase in EPG, which may result in part from increased gluconeogenesis in the liver and kidneys. Glucose utilization is down-regulated, while increased lipid responses, involving lipolysis, lipid oxidation and ketogenesis, increase markedly after SGLT2 inhibitor treatment. Elevated levels of ketone bodies may serve as an additional energy substrate, improving heart and kidney performance. Protein catabolism may also be involved in the metabolic adaptation process during SGLT2 treatment. BCAAs are derived from skeletal muscle or dietary proteins and are then used in myocardial and renal cells to meet the needs of energy metabolism. Increased protein catabolism, together with increased lipolysis, ultimately leads to loss of body weight, including lean and fat mass, contributing to improved b-cell function and insulin sensitivity. Abbreviations: SGLT2: sodium-glucose co-transporter 2; GLP-1: glucagon-like peptide-1; TCA: tricarboxylic acid cycle; mTORC1: mechanistic target of rapamycin complex 1; FFA: free fatty acid; EPG: endogenous glucose production; LV: left ventricle; BCAA: branched-chain amino acid.

2. SGLT2 inhibitors induce a transcriptional paradigm of nutrient deprivation

2.1. Activation of the AMPK/SIRT1/PGC-1a signaling pathway.

As mentioned above, SGLT2 inhibition results in a net caloric loss, which mimics a metabolic paradigm as during fasting and thus induces the nutrient deprivation pathway. In a series of experimental studies, SGLT2 inhibitors have been shown to activate the AMPK/SIRT1/PGC-1a signaling pathway, thereby increasing fatty acid oxidation, gluconeogenesis and ketogenesis, mimicking a fasting-like metabolic state and remarkably ameliorating the energy deficit state (108,109).

More importantly, activation of the AMPK/SIRT1/PGC-1a signaling pathway induced by SGLT2 inhibition, will also ameliorate mitochondrial dysfunction, thus attenuating oxidative stress, endoplasmic reticulum (ER) stress, inflammation and apoptosis (110).

In addition, the AMPK/SIRT1/PGC-1a pathway activated by SGLT2 inhibition may exert further pleiotropic cardioprotective effects. The nutrient-sensing pathway induced by SGLT2 inhibition enhances autophagy in the heart and kidneys.

Autophagy-mediated recycling of cellular components may explain the restoration of ATP production and reduction of oxidative stress (111).

Furthermore, activation of the AMPK/SIRT1/PGC-1a pathway has been reported to tightly modulate hypoxia-inducible factor (HIF) in diabetes-related kidney damage ; given that the increase in hematocrit after SGLT2 inhibitor treatment was considered to account for ≈50% of the cardiovascular benefit of major adverse cardiovascular events in the EMPA-REG OUTCOME study, the cardioprotection induced by SGLT2 inhibitors could be partly due to their erythropoietic effects (112).

Further studies are needed to elucidate the effects and molecular mechanisms of SGLT2 inhibition in order to better clarify the cardio-renal protective mechanisms of SGLT2 inhibitors.

2.2. Inhibition of the mTOR signaling pathway

mTOR is a serine/threonine kinase complex; there are two distinct mTOR complexes: mTORC1 and mTORC2; mTORC1 is considered a nutrient sensor responsible for stimulating anabolic metabolism for cell growth and proliferation, and inhibits autophagy (113). Overactivation of mTORC1 has been reported to lead to dysfunction and adverse cardiac remodeling (114) as well as renal dysfunction, albuminuria and interstitial fibrosis (115).

In a series of experimental studies, SGLT2 inhibitors inhibited the mTOR signalling pathway and maintained redox homeostasis, regulated autophagy and suppressed inflammation, which may explain the cardio-renal protection of SGLT2 (116-118). Furthermore, using a mouse model with diabetic nephropathy, Tomita et al. (119) reported that ATP production in proximal epithelial tubular cells shifted from lipolysis to ketolysis, and that treatment with Empagliflozin restored ATP levels in the kidney and ameliorated renal damage.

High levels of ketone bodies were also shown to attenuate mTORC1-associated tubular epithelial cell damage in mice with non-proteinuric diabetic kidney disease and podocyte damage in diabetic mice, establishing a novel link between SGLT2 inhibition, ketone bodies, mTOR signaling and renal protection. To date, the detailed molecular mechanisms by which SGLT2 inhibitors contribute to increased ketone body levels, as well as the mechanisms underlying elevated ketone body utilization in damaged kidneys, remain unresolved; further research is needed to answer these questions.

In summary, metabolic reprogramming plays an important role in the progression of heart failure and diabetic nephropathy; SGLT2 inhibitors trigger metabolic readjustments in the context of heart failure and diabetic kidney disease, which may partly explain the mechanisms of their cardio-renal protective effects; SGLT2 inhibition leads to marked glycosuria and net caloric loss, mimicking a fasting-type metabolic response. Energy substrates shift from carbohydrates to GAs and ketone bodies, restoring ATP levels; in addition, SGLT2 inhibitors induce a transcriptional paradigm of nutrient deprivation by acting on nutrient-sensing pathways, involving the AMPK/SIRT1/PGC-1a and mTOR pathways, leading to improved mitochondrial function, insulin resistance, inflammation, oxidative stress and enhanced autophagy, thus contributing to cardio-renal protection. The mechanisms of action of SGLT2 inhibitors in cardio-renal protection based on metabolic reprogramming are shown in Figure 4.

VII. Effects of SGLT2 inhibitors on non-diabetic patients with chronic kidney disease (DAPA-CKD trial)

To date, three major cardiovascular prognostic trials have demonstrated the beneficial effects of these agents beyond glycemic control (61,120,121). These trials enrolled patients with type 2 diabetes and established cardiovascular disease or cardiovascular risk factors. All three trials reported preservation of renal function (61,120,121).

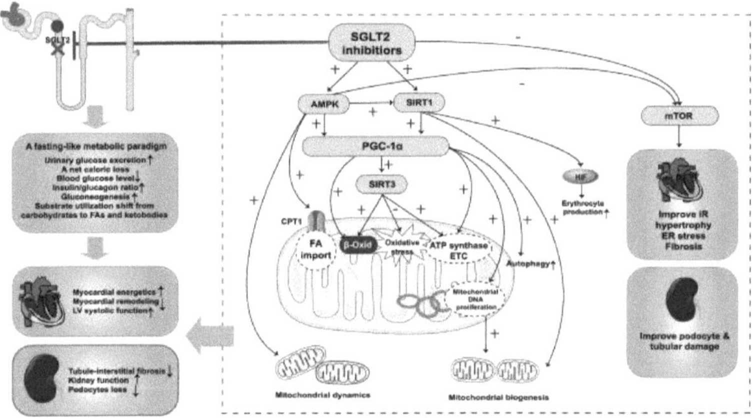

Fig. 4: Cardio-renal protection of SGLT2 inhibitors based on metabolic reprogramming.

Inhibition of SGLT2 results in marked glycosuria and net caloric loss, mimicking a fasting-type metabolic response. Energy substrates shift from carbohydrates to fatty acids and ketone bodies, which restore ATP levels to exert cardiorenal protective effects. SGLT2 inhibitors induce a transcriptional paradigm of nutrient deprivation by acting on nutrient-sensing pathways. SGLT2 inhibitors activate the AMPK/SIRT1/PGC-1a pathway, enhancing FAO and ketogenesis, thereby improving the energy status of the heart and kidneys. In addition, the activated AMPK/SIRT1/PGC-1a pathway exerts other protective effects, including enhancing mitochondrial biogenesis and dynamics, strengthening autophagy and attenuating oxidative stress. SGLT2 inhibitors inhibit the mTOR pathway and thus improve insulin resistance, cardiac hypertrophy, fibrosis and oxidative stress. In addition, inhibition of mTORC1 prevents tubular and podocyte damage, partly through the effects of increased ketone bodies on mTORC1. Abbreviations: SGLT2: sodium-glucose co-transporter 2; FA: fatty acids; LV: left ventricular; mTOR: mechanistic target of rapamycin; mTORC1: mechanistic target of rapamycin complex 1; SIRT1: silent information regulator 1; PGC-1a: peroxisome proliferator-activated receptor-gamma co-activator 1a; SIRT3: silent information regulator 3, HIF: hypoxia-inducible factor; CPT-1: carnitine palmitoyl transferase-1; b-Oxid: b-oxidation; ATP: adenosine triphosphate; ETC: electron transfer chain; DNA: deoxyribonucleic acid; IR: insulin resistance; ER: endoplasmic reticulum. Electron transfer chain; DNA: deoxyribonucleic acid; IR: insulin resistance; ER: endoplasmic reticulum.

However, the lower proportion of participants with chronic kidney disease (CKD) and the smaller number of patients with end-stage renal disease (ESRD) highlighted the need for specific outcome trials to determine the efficacy and safety of SGLT2 in patients with established CKD. The first trial of SGLT2 inhibition included patients with type 2 diabetes and CKD, and reported that canagliflozin 100 mg/day reduced the risk of a composite renal endpoint (including doubling of serum creatinine, ESRD or death from renal or cardiovascular disease) by 30% compared with placebo (122). In the cardiovascular and renal outcome trials mentioned above, the nephroprotective effects of SGLT2 inhibitors do not appear to be fully explained by modest reductions in HbA1c, which are attenuated in patients with low estimated glomerular filtration rate (eGFR). Other beneficial mechanisms, including activation of glomerulotubular feedback and reduction of intrarenal hypoxia, have been proposed to explain the beneficial effects of SGLT2 inhibitors on renal function; these mechanisms may be relevant to CKD in non-diabetic patients (123,124). The Dapagliflozin and Prevention of Adverse Outcomes in CKD (DAPA-CKD) tested the hypothesis that treatment with dapagliflozin was superior to placebo in reducing the risk of renal and cardiovascular events in CKD patients (with and without concomitant type 2 diabetes) who received optimized doses of angiotensin-converting enzyme (ACE) inhibitors or angiotensin receptor blockers (ARBs) as background renoprotective therapy.

1. Aim of the study

The primary objective of the DAPA-CKD trial was to assess whether dapagliflozin reduced the composite endpoint of worsening renal function (defined as a composite endpoint of >50% decrease in eGFR, ESRD or renal death) or cardiovascular death in patients with CKD compared with placebo. In addition, the trial will examine the effect of dapagliflozin versus placebo on the composite endpoint of worsening renal function, the composite endpoint of hospitalization for heart failure or cardiovascular death, and all-cause mortality. Other exploratory endpoints included changes in eGFR and urinary albumin/creatinine ratio (UACR), and health-related quality of life. This study is registered at www.clinicaltrials.gov (NCT03036150).

2. Overall study design

DAPA-CKD is a multinational, multicenter, randomized, double-blind, parallel-group, placebo-controlled study that will recruit 4,300 patients at nearly 400 sites in 21 countries (Figure 5). Figure 6 shows the overall design of the study.

3. Trial participants

Trial participants are adults with CKD with eGFR ≥ 25 but ≤ 75 ml/min/1.73 m^2 and UACR ≥ 200 mg/g but ≤ to 5000 mg/g (≥ 22.6 but ≤ to 565 mg/mmol). Further inclusion and exclusion criteria are listed in Table 2.

4. Statistical considerations

Sample size calculation: DAPA-CKD is an event-driven study. The sample size was based on the expected incidence of the primary efficacy endpoint and the expected effect size of dapagliflozin treatment. After enrolling at least 4,000 patients, the trial had 90% power to detect a 22% relative risk reduction for the primary endpoint, based on primary events observed in 681 patients and a two-sided P value of 0.05. Assumptions for sample size calculation included a placebo event rate of 7.5% per year (based on event rates observed in relevant patients in previous trials), a drug discontinuation rate of 6% per year, a loss to follow-up of 1%, and a recruitment period of 24 months, with a total study duration of 45 months.

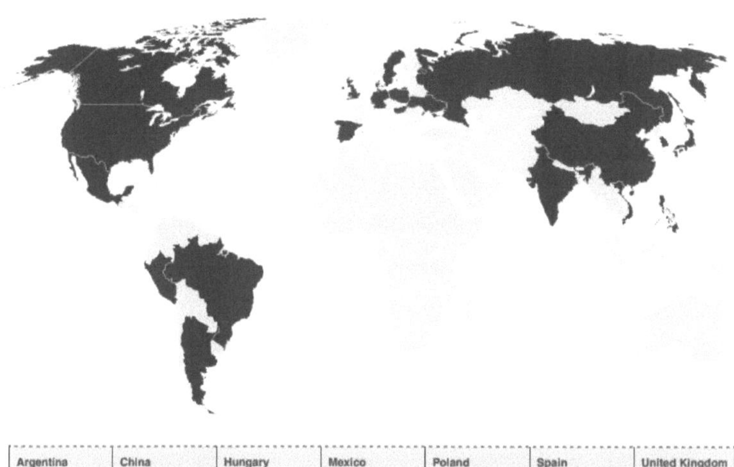

Argentina	China	Hungary	Mexico	Poland	Spain	United Kingdom
Brazil	Denmark	India	Peru	Russia	Sweden	United States
Canada	Germany	Japan	Philippines	South Korea	Ukraine	Vietnam

FIGURE 5: Countries participating in the DAPA-CKD program. H.J.L. Heerspink et al. (125).

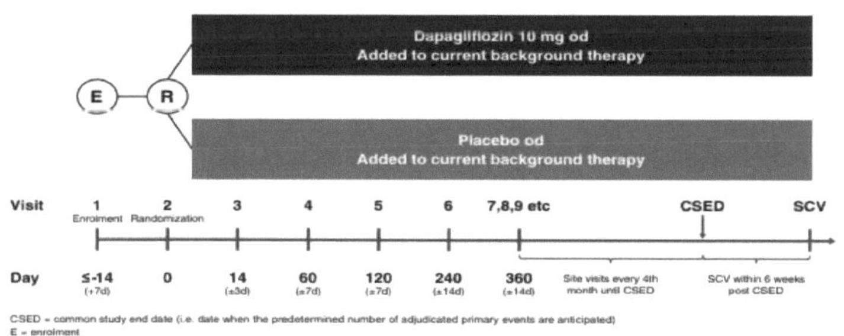

FIGURE 6: Schematic diagram of the DAPA-CKD study. H.J.L. Heerspink et al. (125).

Table 2. Main inclusion and exclusion criteria for the DAPA-CKD trial

Critères d'inclusion

- âgé ≥ 18 ans

- DFGe de ≥25 et ≤ 75 ml/min/1,73 m2 au moment du dépistage

- UACR de ≥200 et ≤ 5000 mg/g au moment du dépistage

- Stabilité et, pour le patient, dose maximale tolérée d'un IEC ou d'un ARA pendant au moins 4 semaines avant la sélection s'il n'y a pas de contre-indication médicale.

Critères d'exclusion

- Diabète sucré de type 1

- Maladie rénale polykystique autosomique dominante ou autosomique récessive, néphrite lupique ou vascularite associée aux ANCA

- Traitement cytotoxique, immunosuppresseur ou autre immunothérapie pour une maladie rénale primaire ou secondaire dans les 6 mois avant l'inscription

- Insuffisance cardiaque congestive de classe IV de la New York Heart Association

- Infarctus du myocarde, angor instable, accident vasculaire cérébral ou accident ischémique transitoire dans les 8 semaines précédant l'inscription.

- Revascularisation coronarienne (intervention coronarienne percutanée ou pontage aorto-coronarien) ou réparation/remplacement valvulaire dans les 8 semaines avant l'inscription

- Toute affection en dehors de la zone d'étude rénale et cardiovasculaire avec une espérance de vie <2 ans sur la base des données de l'étude selon le jugement clinique de l'investigateur

- Insuffisance hépatique [transaminase aspartate ou transaminase alanine >3 fois la limite supérieure de la normale (LSN) ou bilirubine totale >2 fois la LSN au moment de l'inscription.

5. Results

5.1. Participants and follow-up

From February 2017 to October 2018, a total of 7517 participants were selected, of whom 4094 were randomly assigned. Due to regulatory delays, recruitment in China did not begin until December 2019, after which 210 Chinese participants were randomly assigned until March 2020. Baseline characteristics, including medications for type 2 diabetes and renal disease, were balanced between the dapagliflozin and placebo groups (Table 3). Mean age (±ET) was 61.8±12.1 years, 1425 Participants (33.1%) were women. Estimated mean GFR was 43.1±12.4 ml per minute per 1.73 m², median urinary albumin/creatinine ratio was 949 and 2906 participants (67.5%) were diagnosed with type 2 diabetes.

Following a regular meeting on March 26, 2020, the independent Data Monitoring Committee recommended that the two co-principal investigators (first and last author) discontinue the trial due to evidence of efficacy, based on 408 primary endpoint outcome events. The trial management team has accepted this recommendation and selected April 3, 2020 as the cut-off date for all efficacy analyses.

At the end of the trial, median follow-up was 2.4 years (interquartile range 2.0 to 2.7). For reasons other than death, 274 (12.7%) participants discontinued dapagliflozin and 309 (14.4%) participants discontinued placebo. A total of 4,289 participants (99.7%) completed the trial (i.e. were alive and had follow-up data available at the end-of-trial visit, or died during follow-up). A total of 11 participants (0.3%) withdrew their consent, and all but 5 participants (0.3%) were monitored for vital status.

5.2. Efficiency result

The primary composite endpoint of a sustained eGFR reduction of at least 50%, end-stage renal failure or renal or cardiovascular death occurred in 197 subjects (9.2%) in the dapagliflozin arm and 312 subjects (14.5%) in the placebo arm (HR: 0.61; 95% confidence interval [CI], 0.51 to 0.72; P<0.001) (Table 4 and Figure 7A). Event rates for all components of the combined results support dapagliflozin (Table 4). The number of participants who required treatment to prevent a primary outcome event during the trial was 19 (95% CI, 15 to 27). The effect of dapagliflozin on the primary outcome was generally consistent across the predefined subgroups. Among participants with type 2 diabetes, the proportional hazard (HR) for the comparison of the primary endpoint of

Table 3: Demographic and clinical characteristics of participants at baseline in the DAPA-CKD trial.* H. J.L. Heerspink (61)

Characteristic	Dapagliflozin (N=2152)	Placebo (N=2152)
Age — yr	61.8±12.1	61.9±12.1
Female sex — no. (%)	709 (32.9)	716 (33.3)
Race — no. (%)†		
White	1124 (52.2)	1166 (54.2)
Black	104 (4.8)	87 (4.0)
Asian	749 (34.8)	718 (33.4)
Other	175 (8.1)	181 (8.4)
Weight — kg	81.5±20.1	82.0±20.9
Body-mass index‡	29.4±6.0	29.6±6.3
Current smoker — no. (%)	283 (13.2)	301 (14.0)
Blood pressure — mm Hg		
Systolic	136.7±17.5	137.4±17.3
Diastolic	77.5±10.7	77.5±10.3
Estimated GFR		
Mean — ml/min/1.73 m^2	43.2±12.3	43.0±12.4
Distribution — no. (%)		
≥60 ml/min/1.73 m^2	234 (10.9)	220 (10.2)
45 to <60 ml/min/1.73 m^2	646 (30.0)	682 (31.7)
30 to <45 ml/min/1.73 m^2	979 (45.5)	919 (42.7)
<30 ml/min/1.73 m^2	293 (13.6)	331 (15.4)
Hemoglobin — g/liter	128.6±18.1	127.9±18.0
Serum potassium — mEq/liter	4.6±0.5	4.6±0.6
Urinary albumin-to-creatinine ratio§		
Median (interquartile range)	965 (472–1903)	934 (482–1868)
>1000 — no. (%)	1048 (48.7)	1031 (47.9)
Type 2 diabetes — no. (%)	1455 (67.6)	1451 (67.4)
Cardiovascular disease — no. (%)¶	813 (37.8)	797 (37.0)
Heart failure — no. (%)	235 (10.9)	233 (10.8)
Previous medication — no. (%)		
ACE inhibitor	673 (31.3)	681 (31.6)
ARB	1444 (67.1)	1426 (66.3)
Diuretic	928 (43.1)	954 (44.3)
Statin	1395 (64.8)	1399 (65.0)

† Race reported by surveyors; "other" designation includes Native Hawaiian or other Pacific Islander, American Indian or Alaska Native, and other.

‡ Body mass index is weight in kilograms divided by the square of height in meters.

§ The albumin/creatinine ratio was calculated from albumin measured in milligrams and creatinine measured in grams.

¶ Cardiovascular disease was defined as a history of peripheral arterial disease, angina pectoris, myocardial infarction, percutaneous coronary intervention, coronary artery bypass grafting, heart failure, valvular heart disease, abdominal aortic aneurysm, atrial fibrillation, atrial flutter, ischemic stroke, transient ischemic attack, hemorrhagic stroke, carotid artery stenosis, pacemaker insertion, stenting, coronary artery stenosis, ventricular arrhythmia, implantable cardioverter-defibrillator, non-coronary revascularization or surgical amputation.

dapagliflozin versus placebo was 0.64 (95% CI, 0.52 to 0.79), versus 0.50 (95% CI, 0.35 to 0.72) for non-diabetic type 2 patients.

The incidence of each secondary outcome was lower in the dapagliflozin group than in the placebo group (Table 4). The proportional hazard HR for the composite renal outcome of sustained eGFR decline of at least 50%, end-stage renal failure or renal death was 0.56 (95% CI, 0.45 to 0.68; P < 0.001) (Table 4 and Figure 7B). The HR for the composite endpoint of death from cardiovascular causes or hospitalization for heart failure was 0.71 (95% CI, 0.55 to 0.92; P = 0.009) (Table 4 and Figure 7C). There were 101 (4.7%) all-cause deaths in the dapagliflozin group and 146 (6.8%) all-cause deaths in the placebo group (HR: 0.69; 95% CI, 0.53 to 0.88; P = 0.004) (Table 4 and Figure 7D).

5.3. Safety results and adverse events

The rates of adverse events and serious adverse events were generally similar in the dapagliflozin and placebo groups (Table 4). Participants who received dapagliflozin reported no episodes of diabetic ketoacidosis, an event observed in two participants who received placebo. No diabetic ketoacidosis or severe hypoglycemia was observed in participants without type 2 diabetes. There was one confirmed case of Fournier's gangrene in the placebo group, but none in the dapagliflozin group.

Outcome	Dapagliflozin		Placebo		Hazard Ratio (95% CI)	P Value
	no./total no. (%)	*events/100 patient-yr*	*no./total no. (%)*	*events/100 patient-yr*		
Primary outcome						
Primary composite outcome	197/2152 (9.2)	4.6	312/2152 (14.5)	7.5	0.61 (0.51–0.72)	<0.001
Decline in estimated GFR of ≥50%	112/2152 (5.2)	2.6	201/2152 (9.3)	4.8	0.53 (0.42–0.67)	NA
End-stage kidney disease	109/2152 (5.1)	2.5	161/2152 (7.5)	3.8	0.64 (0.50–0.82)	NA
Estimated GFR of <15 ml/min/1.73 m^2	84/2152 (3.9)	1.9	120/2152 (5.6)	2.8	0.67 (0.51–0.88)	NA
Long-term dialysis†	68/2152 (3.2)	1.5	99/2152 (4.6)	2.2	0.66 (0.48–0.90)	NA
Kidney transplantation†	3/2152 (0.1)	0.1	8/2152 (0.4)	0.2	—	NA
Death from renal causes	2/2152 (<0.1)	0.0	6/2152 (0.3)	0.1	—	NA
Death from cardiovascular causes	65/2152 (3.0)	1.4	80/2152 (3.7)	1.7	0.81 (0.58–1.12)	NA
Secondary outcomes						
Composite of decline in estimated GFR of ≥50%, end-stage kidney disease, or death from renal causes	142/2152 (6.6)	3.3	243/2152 (11.3)	5.8	0.56 (0.45–0.68)	<0.001
Composite of death from cardiovascular causes or hospitalization for heart failure	100/2152 (4.6)	2.2	138/2152 (6.4)	3.0	0.71 (0.55–0.92)	0.009
Death from any cause	101/2152 (4.7)	2.2	146/2152 (6.8)	3.1	0.69 (0.53–0.88)	0.004
Safety outcomes‡						
Discontinuation of regimen due to adverse event	118/2149 (5.5)	—	123/2149 (5.7)	—	—	0.79
Any serious adverse event	633/2149 (29.5)	—	729/2149 (33.9)	—	—	0.002
Adverse events of interest						
Amputation§	35/2149 (1.6)	—	39/2149 (1.8)	—	—	0.73
Any definite or probable diabetic ketoacidosis	0/2149	—	2/2149 (<0.1)	—	—	0.50
Fracture¶	85/2149 (4.0)	—	69/2149 (3.2)	—	—	0.22
Renal-related adverse event¶	155/2149 (7.2)	—	188/2149 (8.7)	—	—	0.07
Major hypoglycemia‖	14/2149 (0.7)	—	28/2149 (1.3)	—	—	0.04
Volume depletion¶	127/2149 (5.9)	—	90/2149 (4.2)	—	—	0.01

Tableau 4 : Résultats primaires et secondaires et évènements indésirables d'intérêt particulier. H. J.L. Heerspink (50) térêparticulier*. H. J.L. Heerspink (50) particulier*. Résultats primaires et secondaires et événements indésirables d'intérêt particulier

* NA means not applicable, as P values for efficacy outcomes are only reported for outcomes that have been included in the hierarchical test strategy.

† For the long-term dialysis or kidney transplant composite, there were 69 outcome events in the dapagliflozin group and 100 outcome events in the placebo group (hazard ratio, 0.66; 95% CI, 0.49 to 0.90).

‡ Safety analyses included all randomized participants who received at least one dose of dapagliflozin or placebo.

§ These results are based on a predefined list of preferred terms.

‖ The following criteria were confirmed by the investigator: symptoms of severe disturbance of consciousness or behavior, need for outside help, intervention to treat hypoglycemia, and rapid recovery from acute symptoms after intervention.

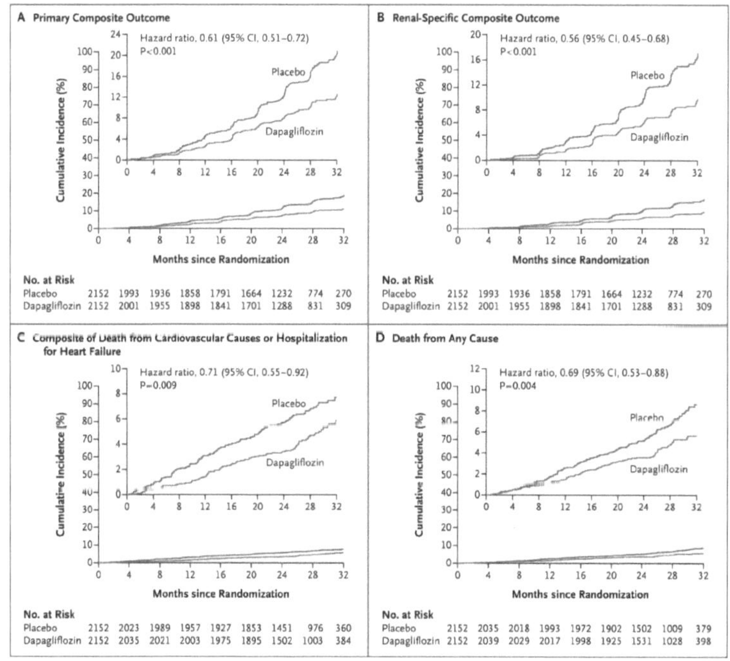

Figure 7: Primary and secondary results of the DAPA-CKD study. H. J.L. Heerspink (61)

6. Discussion

SGLT2 inhibitors have become effective drugs for reducing the incidence of renal and cardiovascular events in patients with type 2 diabetes. Their apparent ability to slow the progressive decline in renal function over time cannot be fully explained by improved glycemic control involving other non-glycemic pathways. These include natriuretic/osmotic diuresis, restoration of tubulo-glomerular feedback control leading to glomerular afferent vasoconstriction and reduction of individual nephron hyperfiltration, amelioration of renal tissue hypoxia and reduction of inflammation and fibrosis (123,126). SGLT2 inhibitors may also be beneficial in non-diabetic CKD patients if one or more of these mechanisms are involved. DAPA-CKD will test this hypothesis by evaluating whether dapagliflozin safely reduces the risk of combined renal and cardiovascular disease. Risk of the composite endpoint of renal and cardiovascular mortality in a wide range of diabetic and non-diabetic CKD patients already receiving optimized standard nephroprotective therapy.

The likely efficacy and safety of dapagliflozin in CKD and non-diabetic patients was an important consideration in the design of the DAPA-CKD study. In previous studies, some non-diabetic patients had been exposed to SGLT2 inhibitors. All these previous studies have shown that SGLT2 inhibition induces glycosuria and results in lower blood pressure, body weight and uricemia (127,128). Hypoglycemia is a particular safety concern for most hypoglycemic drugs. However, glycosuria induced by SGLT2 inhibitors was reduced with decreasing blood glucose concentrations and filtered glucose load, which explains why hypoglycemia is not an inherent risk of these drugs. In addition, compensatory increases in basal hepatic glucose production following urinary glucose loss help to maintain fasting blood glucose at euglycemic levels in non-diabetic individuals (129). Moreover, in patients with CKD, due to reduced glomerular glucose filtration, the load of filtered glucose is also reduced. It is therefore not surprising that in a pooled analysis of randomized controlled trials in patients with type 2 diabetes with an eGFR of 15-45 ml/min/1.73 m^2, the incidence of hypoglycemia was similar (130).

We are collecting additional specific safety data related to hypoglycemic therapy in general and SGLT2 inhibitors in particular, including information on bone fractures, diabetic ketoacidosis, amputations and acute kidney injury (AKI). AKI is of particular interest in the treatment of DAPA-CKD because the hemodynamic effects of SGLT2 inhibitors can lead to an initial decrease in eGFR similar to that seen with ACE inhibitors or ARBs, although this is due to a different blood hemodynamic mechanism (i.e. constriction of afferent arterioles with SGLT2 inhibitors and dilation of efferent arterioles with renin-angiotensin system inhibitors) (131). Despite these similarities, fewer episodes of ARF were reported with SGLT2 inhibition in the Effects of Dapagliflozin on Cardiovascular Events-Thrombolysis in Myocardial Infarction 58 (DECLARE-TIMI 58) programs, Empagliflozin Abolishes Cardiovascular Excess Glycemia in Type 2 Diabetes SGLT2 Inhibition Reported Fewer AKI Episodes in the Outcome Events Trial (EMPA-REG) Program (OUTCOME), Canagliflozin Cardiovascular Assessment Study (CANVAS) and Canagliflozin and Renal Endpoints in Diabetic Nephropathy Clinical Evaluation (CREDENCE). Although these results are based on investigator-reported adverse events, they were not specifically defined or evaluated by these investigators (16,120-122). To properly determine the effect of dapagliflozin on AKI in patients with CKD, all potentially severe AKI (defined as a doubling of serum creatinine compared with the last core laboratory measurement) were evaluated by an independent investigator. An unexpected increase in lower-limb amputation rates with canagliflozin was reported in the CANVAS study but not in the CREDENCE trial (121,122). This phenomenon was not observed with dapagliflozin in any of the previous studies, including DECLARE-TIMI 58 and dapagliflozin and the prevention of adverse outcomes in heart failure (DAPA-HF), and in the EMPA-REG OUTCOME study, Empagliflozin did not observe this phenomenon (16,120). However, regulations require that all amputations and events leading to an increased risk of amputation be collected from all ongoing trials of SGLT2 inhibitors, including DAPA-CKD.

From an efficacy perspective, DAPA-CKD will determine the effect of dapagliflozin on the composite renal endpoint that has been used in previous chronic kidney disease trials. The most clinically significant component of this endpoint was end-stage renal disease, defined as initiation of dialysis for more than 28 days or renal transplantation. A sustained eGFR <15 ml/min/1.73 m^2 is also included in the definition of ESRD. This measure was considered clinically relevant given the increased risk of death and reduced quality of life in people with an eGFR below 15 ml/min/1.73 m^2. A >50% decrease in eGFR, which corresponds to an 80% increase in serum creatinine, is an additional component, in contrast to other trials that used a doubling of serum creatinine or a >40% decrease as the eGFR component of a composite renal endpoint (132).

We decided not to use the >40% reduction in eGFR because dapagliflozin can cause an acute reduction in eGFR with a hemodynamic component. This can potentially lead to eGFR reductions of up to 40%, which do not reflect the true progression of chronic kidney disease, diminishing the ability to differentiate between placebo and dapagliflozin and increasing the risk of a Type 1 error (T. Greene, submitted for publication). A doubling of serum creatinine was not considered, as a >50% reduction in eGFR was found to be an equally robust measure of a significant decline in renal function and would likely reduce sample size and complexity of test performance. The primary endpoint also included renal or cardiovascular death. All-cause mortality was not included, because dapagliflozin is unlikely to affect deaths not related to renal or cardiovascular causes.

How do participants in the DAPA-CKD trial compare with those enrolled in other SGLT2 inhibitor trials? A small number of patients enrolled in the SGLT2 Inhibitor Cardiovascular Outcomes Trial had CKD as defined by eGFR or UACR. CREDENCE is the only trial to date to have recruited only patients with type 2 diabetes and CKD. In the DAPA-CKD study, 90% of patients had an eGFR < 60 ml/min/1.73 m^2 and at least 80% of participants had a UACR > 300 mg/g (Figure 8). Given that low eGFR and high UACR are important risk markers for renal and cardiovascular events, cardiovascular event rates in DAPA-CKD are expected to be at least comparable to those in the ISGLT2 cardiovascular outcomes study. In comparing DAPA-CKD with two other SGLT2 renal outcome trials (CREDENCE and EMPA-KIDNEY), DAPA-CKD will include a broader population than CREDENCE; the latter only included patients with type 2 diabetes (Figure 9). The EMPA-KIDNEY trial, which evaluated empagliflozin versus placebo, further expanded the inclusion criteria to include patients with type 1 diabetes and UACR <200 mg/g (if eGFR between 20 and 45 ml/min/1.73 m^2) (Figure 9).
Taken together, these three trials will help determine the optimal use of SGLT2 inhibitors in the treatment of CKD.

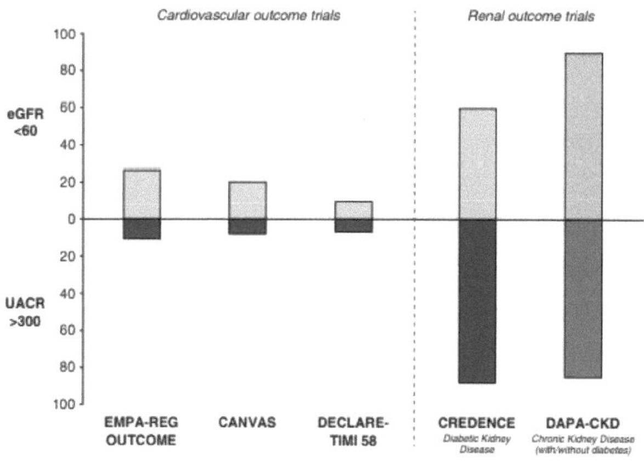

Figure 8: Proportion of patients with eGFR <60 ml/min/1.73 m2 and UACR ≥300 mg/g in completed SGLT2 inhibitor trials versus DAPA-CKD. DAPA-

CKD interim reference data (data stopped in September 2019) were used to create the figure. H.J.L. Heerspink et al. (125).

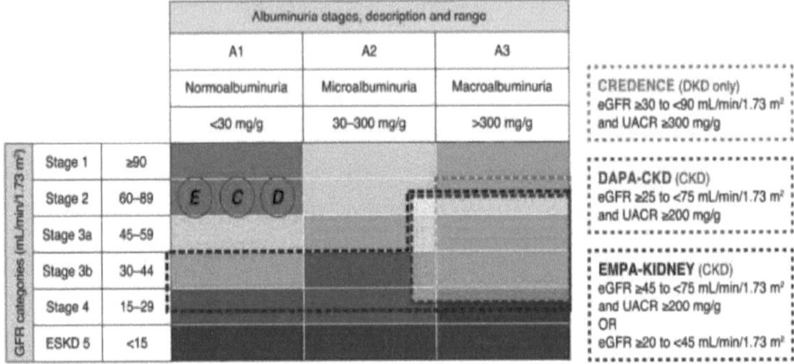

Figure 9: National Kidney Foundation classification of chronic kidney disease. The range of UACR and eGFR for inclusion in the CREDENCE (green), DAPA-CKD (blue) and EMPA-KIDNEY (purple) trials is shown. The white shaded area indicates the eGFR and UACR inclusion criteria in the DAPA-CKD trial. Cardiovascular outcome trials are shown in circles and positioned according to their mean eGFR and median UACR. H.J.L. Heerspink et al. (125).

During the DAPA-CKD trial, the results of two other major cardiovascular outcome trials with dapagliflozin, DECLARE-TIMI 58 and DAPA-HF, were also presented.

The DECLARE-TIMI 58 trial reported that in type 2 diabetic patients with predominantly preserved renal function and with or at risk of cardiovascular disease, dapagliflozin significantly reduced the composite endpoint rate of heart failure or cardiovascular death by 17%, and the composite endpoint risk of >40% eGFR decline, ESRD and renal death by 47% (120). The DAPA-HF study showed that in patients with reduced ejection fraction heart failure, with or without type 2 diabetes, dapagliflozin significantly reduced the risk of heart failure or cardiovascular death (133). These effects were remarkably consistent in patients with and without type 2 diabetes, and in patients with and without CKD. In addition, the trial reported that the rate of renal-related serious adverse events was significantly lower in the dapagliflozin group (1.6%) than in the placebo group (2.7%; P = 0.009). These results are promising for patients with chronic renal failure, but need to be confirmed by DAPA-CKD studies.

In conclusion, the DAPA-CKD study is the first clinical trial dedicated to exploring the potential benefits and risks of SGLT2 inhibitors in patients at different stages of CKD (with or without diabetes) who have received renoprotective therapy.

VIII. Renal, cardiovascular and safety outcomes of canagliflozin according to baseline renal function: CREDENCE randomized trial

Despite the reduced efficacy of canagliflozin in lowering blood glucose levels in patients with renal failure, the interest in investigating the renoprotective effects of canagliflozin in the CREDENCE (Clinical Evaluation of Canagliflozin and Renal Events in Patients with Diabetic Kidney Disease) trial was based on the following findings: favorable effects on reduction of urinary albumin/creatinine ratio (UACR) and preservation of eGFR were observed in early glycemic control studies (126,134). The acute and modest decrease in eGFR observed in earlier studies attenuated over time and is consistent with the hemodynamic effects observed with angiotensin-converting enzyme inhibitors and angiotensin receptor blockers (135).

The strong correlation between albuminuria and renal clinical outcomes, and the idea that these drugs could reduce intra-glomerular pressure, led to the hypothesis that they could prevent the progression of diabetic nephropathy, including in people with low eGFR, possibly linked to the hypoglycemic effect. The CREDENCE study was designed to assess the benefit of canagliflozin on the risk of renal failure and cardiovascular events in type 2 diabetic patients at high risk of disease progression, while also evaluating its safety.

Canagliflozin safely reduced renal and cardiovascular events in the CREDENCE study population (122). In a secondary analysis of the CREDENCE study, we investigated whether the effects of canagliflozin on clinically important renal, cardiovascular and safety outcomes were consistent across the wide range of eGFRs included, including the 30-45 ml/min per 1.73 m^2 GFR range where the glycemic effect is smallest.

1. Methods

CREDENCE is a multicenter, randomized, double-blind, placebo-controlled clinical trial evaluating the effects of canagliflozin on clinically important renal, cardiovascular and safety parameters in patients with type 2 diabetes and CKD.

1.1. Study participants

Eligible participants were aged ≥30 years and had type 2 diabetes, HbA1c levels between 6.5% and 12.0%, an eGFR between 30 and 90 ml/min per 1.73 m^2 and an ABR between 300 and 5000 mg/g (33,9-565.6 mg/mmol), and received the maximum stable marker or tolerated dose of an angiotensin-converting enzyme inhibitor or angiotensin receptor blocker for 4 weeks prior to randomization. By design, approximately 60% of participants were required to be screened for hypertension. Participants must have an eGFR of 30 to 60 ml/min per 1.73 m^2. Exclusion criteria included non-diabetic nephropathy, type 1 diabetes and previous treatment of nephropathy with an immunosuppressant or a history of renal replacement therapy.

1.2. Randomization, study treatment and eGFR category

Participants were randomized to receive oral canagliflozin 100 mg daily or a matching placebo. The protocol stipulated that study treatment should continue until the onset of dialysis, kidney transplantation, development of diabetic ketoacidosis, pregnancy, receipt of unauthorized treatment or study termination.

Study eligibility criteria included an eGFR of 30-90 ml/min per 1.73 m^2. After screening, participants would continue with a 2-week single-blind placebo trial, or extended screening if necessary for various reasons, including completion of at least 4 weeks of stable-dose renin and angiotensin blockade. Participants who did not enter the two-week run-in period directly had their eGFR remeasured at the start of the run-in period. The most recent eGFR measurement (e.g., at screening or week 22) was taken as the screening eGFR and used to stratify randomization into categories of 30-45, 45-60 and 60-90 ml/min per 1.73 m^2. On the day of randomization, additional baseline eGFR measurements were taken. Background therapy for intensive glycemic management and cardiovascular protection is recommended in accordance with practice guidelines.

1.3. Results

The main result of these analyses was the same as for the main trial (122)Secondary renal outcomes included a composite endpoint of CKD (chronic dialysis ≥30 days, kidney transplant or eGFR<15 ml/min per 1.73 m^2 for a duration ≥30 days, as assessed by the reference laboratory), doubling of serum creatinine from the initial randomized mean value, maintained for ≥30 days, as assessed in the laboratory, or death from renal or cardiovascular disease. Secondary renal outcomes included a composite endpoint of CKD, serum creatinine doubling or renal death; end-stage renal disease; serum creatinine doubling; and an exploratory composite endpoint of RRT initiation (initiation of chronic dialysis ≥30 days or kidney transplant) or renal death.

Other efficacy outcomes included the composite endpoint of cardiovascular death or hospitalization for heart failure; the composite endpoint of cardiovascular death, myocardial infarction or stroke; hospitalization for heart failure; cardiovascular death; and the composite endpoint of cardiovascular death from myocardial infarction, stroke or hospitalization for heart failure or unstable angina. This analysis examined safety events with at least 10 events per eGFR subgroup, including all adverse events and serious adverse events, amputations, fractures, osmotic diuresis and volume depletion.

Renal and cardiovascular outcomes and selected safety endpoints were assessed independently.

1.4. Statistical analysis

The effect of predefined canagliflozin on the primary endpoint was

analyzed in participants with eGFR between 30 and 45, 45 and 60 and 60 and 90 ml/min/1.73 m^2 according to the intention-to-treat approach; analyses of other renal, cardiovascular and safety endpoints were analyzed post hoc. Proportional hazards (HR) and 95% confidence intervals (CI) for all endpoints were estimated using Cox proportional hazards regression. Cox proportional hazards regression models were used in each eGFR stratum. We tested for heterogeneity of treatment effects between screening eGFR categories by adding eGFR categories as a covariate and an interaction term between treatment and eGFR categories to the relevant model.

We calculated the annualized incidence rate per 1000 patient-years of follow-up. The absolute risk difference was calculated by subtracting the number of placebo participants who met the endpoint (per 1000 patients during follow-up) from canagliflozin participants. Heterogeneity in absolute risk reduction for cardiovascular or renal endpoints among eGFR screening subgroups was estimated using fixed-effects meta-analysis. Changes in intermediate outcomes over time for the analysis population during treatment were analyzed using repeated-measures linear mixed-effects models (unless otherwise specified), assuming unstructured covariance and adjusting on the basis of value, test group and test visit. The on-treatment eGFR slope was estimated using all central laboratory eGFR measurements taken between study day 1 and the last dose of study drug, plus 2 days.

The effect of canagliflozin on mean eGFR slope during treatment was analyzed by fitting a two-slope linear mixed-effects spline model (with a node at week 3) to eGFR values with random intercept and random slope treatments. When the unstructured model failed to converge, a simplified model with random intercept and a single random slope was used to account for variation in eGFR trajectories between participants. The overall mean slope was calculated as a weighted combination of the acute and chronic slopes to reflect the mean rate of change in eGFR at week 130. We also provide a visual representation of the pattern of change in mean eGFR using a restricted maximum likelihood repeated measures approach. The analysis included fixed and categorical effects for treatment, visit and treatment-visit interaction, and fixed and continuous covariates for baseline eGFR and baseline eGFR-visit interaction. In the non-randomized subgroup of participants defined by a last-treatment eGFR of <30 ml/min per 1.73 m^2, the number of participants with a first event from the first eGFR <30 ml/min per 1.73 m^2 is summarized below: renal and cardiovascular outcomes. Given the post-hoc nature of many analyses, P-values are presented for descriptive rather than inferential purposes, without adjustment for multiplicity. All analyses were performed using SAS version 9.4.

2. Results

The CREDENCE trial randomized 4401 participants with a median follow-up of 2.62 years (range 0.02-4.53 years), and was stopped for efficacy reasons at an interim analysis, as recommended by the Data Monitoring Committee. At baseline, the mean age of participants was 63 years, 34% were women, 67% were Caucasian and 20% were Asian. Mean HbA1c was 8.3%, mean blood pressure was 140/78 mm Hg, 50% had a history of cardiovascular disease. The mean eGFR at baseline was 56.2

ml/min per 1.73 m^2 and the median UACR was 927 mg/g (105 mg/mmol).

Participants with an eGFR of 30-45, 45-60 and 60-90 ml/min per 1.73 m^2 were 1313 (30%), 1279 (29%) and 1809 (41%), respectively. Baseline characteristics of participants in each eGFR category were balanced between randomization to receive intervention or placebo. Participants with lower eGFR were numerically more likely to be older, to have had diabetes for a longer period, to use more insulin and diuretics, and to have higher levels of proteinuria.

2.1. Renal time-to-event results

The effect of canagliflozin on the primary composite outcome of CKD, doubling of serum creatinine or renal or cardiovascular death (HR, 0.70; 95% CI, 0.59 to 0.82) was unchanged across all eGFR categories (P Interaction= 0.11; Figure 10). Similarly, the effect of canagliflozin on the renal composite score for CKD, doubling of serum creatinine or renal death (HR, 0.66 ; 95% CI, 0.53 to 0.81) and the effect of canagliflozin on CKD, serum creatinine doubling and renal death according to baseline eGFR, RRT initiation or renal death, the results were consistent across all GFR categories with no evidence of a difference in outcome (P interaction >0, 11 for all outcomes). Canagliflozin separately reduced the primary composite endpoint (HR, 0.75; 95% CI, 0.59 to 0.95) and the kidney-specific composite endpoint (HR, 0.71; 95% CI, 0.53 to 0.94) in participants with an eGFR of 30 to 45 ml/min per 1.73 m^2.

2.2. *Cardiovascular* results

Canagliflozin systematically reduced cardiovascular death or stroke.

hospitalizations for heart failure; the composite criterion for cardiovascular deaths, myocardial infarction or stroke;

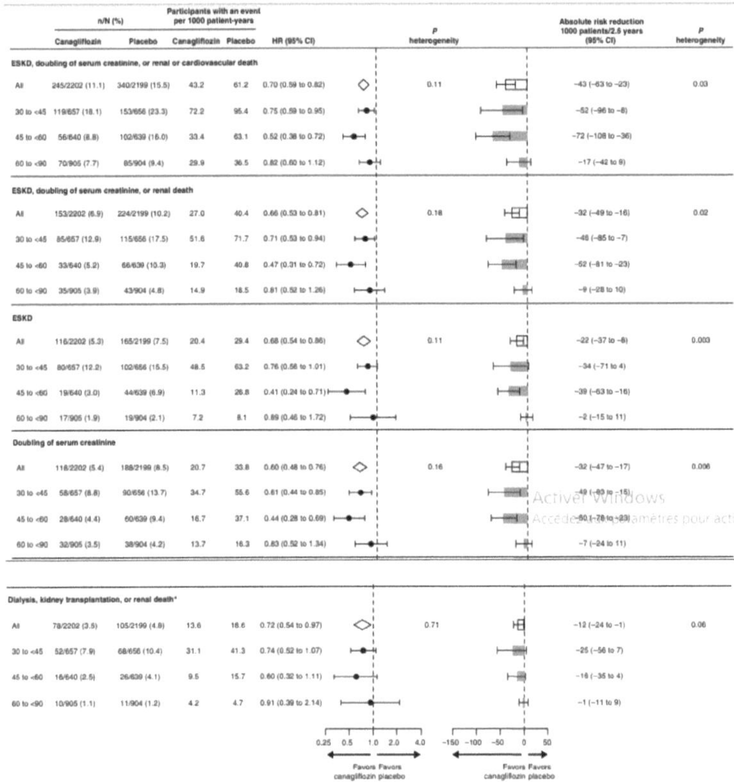

Figure 10: Effect of canagliflozin on renal events. Meg J. Jardine et al., (136).

Canagliflozin reduced renal events in all screening eGFR categories, with greater absolute benefits in the lower categories. * This result was exploratory.

and hospitalization for heart failure in all eGFR subgroups, with all P values for the interaction >0.25 (Figure 11). In particular, canagliflozin reduced the composite endpoint rate of cardiovascular death or hospitalization for heart failure (HR, 0.69; 95% CI, 0.50 to 0.94) in participants with an eGFR of 30 to 45 ml/min per 1.73 m².

	n/N (%)		Participants with an event per 1000 patient-years					
	Canagliflozin	Placebo	Canagliflozin	Placebo	HR (95% CI)	*P* heterogeneity	Absolute risk reduction 1000 patients/2.6 years (95% CI)	*P* heterogeneity
ESKD, doubling of serum creatinine, or renal or cardiovascular death								
All	245/2202 (11.1)	340/2199 (15.5)	43.2	61.2	0.70 (0.59 to 0.82)	0.11	−43 (−63 to −23)	0.03
30 to <45	119/657 (18.1)	153/656 (23.3)	72.2	95.4	0.75 (0.59 to 0.95)		−52 (−96 to −8)	
45 to <60	56/640 (8.8)	102/639 (16.0)	33.4	63.1	0.52 (0.38 to 0.72)		−72 (−108 to −36)	
60 to <90	70/905 (7.7)	85/904 (9.4)	29.9	36.5	0.82 (0.60 to 1.12)		−17 (−42 to 9)	
ESKD, doubling of serum creatinine, or renal death								
All	153/2202 (6.9)	224/2199 (10.2)	27.0	40.4	0.66 (0.53 to 0.81)	0.18	−32 (−49 to −16)	0.02
30 to <45	85/657 (12.9)	115/656 (17.5)	51.6	71.7	0.71 (0.53 to 0.94)		−46 (−85 to −7)	
45 to <60	33/640 (5.2)	66/639 (10.3)	19.7	40.8	0.47 (0.31 to 0.72)		−52 (−81 to −23)	
60 to <90	35/905 (3.9)	43/904 (4.8)	14.9	18.5	0.81 (0.52 to 1.26)		−9 (−28 to 10)	
ESKD								
All	116/2202 (5.3)	165/2199 (7.5)	20.4	29.4	0.68 (0.54 to 0.86)	0.11	−22 (−37 to −8)	0.003
30 to <45	80/657 (12.2)	102/656 (15.5)	48.5	63.2	0.76 (0.56 to 1.01)		−34 (−71 to 4)	
45 to <60	19/640 (3.0)	44/639 (6.9)	11.3	26.8	0.41 (0.24 to 0.71)		−39 (−63 to −16)	
60 to <90	17/905 (1.9)	19/904 (2.1)	7.2	8.1	0.89 (0.46 to 1.72)		−2 (−15 to 11)	
Doubling of serum creatinine								
All	118/2202 (5.4)	188/2199 (8.5)	20.7	33.8	0.60 (0.48 to 0.76)	0.16	−32 (−47 to −17)	0.006
30 to <45	58/657 (8.8)	90/656 (13.7)	34.7	55.6	0.61 (0.44 to 0.85)		−49 (−83 to −15)	
45 to <60	28/640 (4.4)	60/639 (9.4)	16.7	37.1	0.44 (0.28 to 0.69)		−50 (−78 to −23)	
60 to <90	32/905 (3.5)	38/904 (4.2)	13.7	16.3	0.83 (0.52 to 1.34)		−7 (−24 to 11)	
Dialysis, kidney transplantation, or renal death*								
All	78/2202 (3.5)	105/2199 (4.8)	13.8	18.6	0.72 (0.54 to 0.97)	0.71	−12 (−24 to −1)	0.06
30 to <45	52/657 (7.9)	68/656 (10.4)	31.1	41.3	0.74 (0.52 to 1.07)		−25 (−56 to 7)	
45 to <60	16/640 (2.5)	26/639 (4.1)	9.5	15.7	0.60 (0.32 to 1.11)		−16 (−35 to 4)	
60 to <90	10/905 (1.1)	11/904 (1.2)	4.2	4.7	0.91 (0.39 to 2.14)		−1 (−11 to 9)	

Favors canagliflozin Favors placebo

Favors canagliflozin Favors placebo

Figure 11: Effect of canagliflozin on cardiac events. Meg J. Jardine et al. (136).

Canagliflozin reduced cardiovascular outcomes in all eGFR screening categories.

2.3. Security

Overall, canagliflozin resulted in fewer adverse events and serious adverse events, with consistent results in the eGFR screening subgroup (P for interaction=0.40 and 0.15, respectively; Figure 12). Rates of other adverse events, including fractures and amputations, generally did not differ between groups randomized to canagliflozin or placebo, with consistent results in the eGFR subgroups. The exceptions were volume depletion and osmotic dialysis. The exceptions were hypovolemia and osmotic diuresis, which were not significantly more frequent with canagliflozin overall, but there was evidence of differences in effect between eGFR subgroups (P interaction =0.01 and 0.03 respectively). No unexpected safety impact was observed in patients with eGFR between 30-45 ml/min per 1.73 m².

	n/N (%)		Participants with an event per 1000 patient-years			
	Canagliflozin	Placebo	Canagliflozin	Placebo	HR (95%CI)	*P* heterogeneity
Adverse events						
All	1784/2200 (81.1)	1860/2197 (84.7)	351.4	379.3	0.87 (0.82 to 0.93)	0.40
30 to <45	563/655 (86.0)	572/656 (87.2)	394.8	413.5	0.93 (0.83 to 1.05)	
45 to <60	521/640 (81.4)	544/638 (85.3)	345.7	387.7	0.84 (0.74 to 0.95)	
60 to <90	700/905 (77.3)	744/903 (82.4)	326.6	351.4	0.86 (0.77 to 0.95)	
All serious adverse events						
All	737/2200 (33.5)	806/2197 (36.7)	145.2	164.4	0.87 (0.79 to 0.97)	0.15
30 to <45	249/655 (38.0)	283/656 (43.1)	174.6	204.6	0.85 (0.71 to 1.00)	
45 to <60	213/640 (33.3)	249/638 (39.0)	141.3	177.4	0.78 (0.65 to 0.93)	
60 to <90	275/905 (30.4)	274/903 (30.3)	128.3	129.4	0.99 (0.84 to 1.17)	
Amputation						
All	70/2200 (3.2)	63/2197 (2.9)	12.3	11.2	1.11 (0.79 to 1.56)	0.14
30 to <45	23/655 (3.5)	17/656 (2.6)	13.7	10.2	1.36 (0.73 to 2.54)	
45 to <60	15/640 (2.3)	23/638 (3.6)	8.9	14.1	0.64 (0.33 to 1.22)	
60 to <90	32/905 (3.5)	23/903 (2.5)	13.8	9.9	1.40 (0.82 to 2.39)	
Fracture*						
All	67/2200 (3.0)	68/2197 (3.1)	11.8	12.1	0.98 (0.70 to 1.37)	0.77
30 to <45	23/655 (3.5)	22/656 (3.4)	13.7	13.2	1.04 (0.58 to 1.86)	
45 to <60	19/640 (3.0)	23/638 (3.6)	11.4	14.1	0.82 (0.44 to 1.50)	
60 to <90	25/905 (2.8)	23/903 (2.5)	10.7	9.9	1.08 (0.61 to 1.91)	
Osmotic diuresis						
All	51/2200 (2.3)	40/2197 (1.8)	10.0	8.2	1.25 (0.83 to 1.89)	0.03
30 to <45	19/655 (2.9)	15/656 (2.3)	13.3	10.8	1.25 (0.63 to 2.46)	
45 to <60	9/640 (1.4)	16/638 (2.5)	6.0	11.4	0.53 (0.24 to 1.21)	
60 to <90	23/905 (2.5)	9/903 (1.0)	10.7	4.3	2.56 (1.19 to 5.54)	
Volume depletion						
All	144/2200 (6.5)	115/2197 (5.2)	28.4	23.5	1.25 (0.97 to 1.59)	0.01
30 to <45	70/655 (10.7)	36/656 (5.5)	49.1	26.0	1.99 (1.33 to 2.98)	
45 to <60	35/640 (5.5)	36/638 (5.6)	23.2	25.7	0.93 (0.59 to 1.49)	
60 to <90	39/905 (4.3)	43/903 (4.8)	18.2	20.3	0.89 (0.58 to 1.38)	

0.125 0.25 0.5 1.0 2.0 4.0 8.0
Favors canagliflozin Favors placebo

Figure 12: The effect of canagliflozin on safety outcomes. Meg J. Jardine et al. (136). The effect was generally consistent across all eGFR screening categories. *Based on confirmed and adjudicated results.

2.4. Effect on eGFR slope

Canagliflozin resulted in a sharp drop in eGFR at week 3, which was significant in all eGFR subgroups (all P<0.001), although the smallest drop was seen in patients screened for eGFR of 30 to 45 ml/min per 1.73 m² per year (P heterogeneity=0.02); Figure 13).

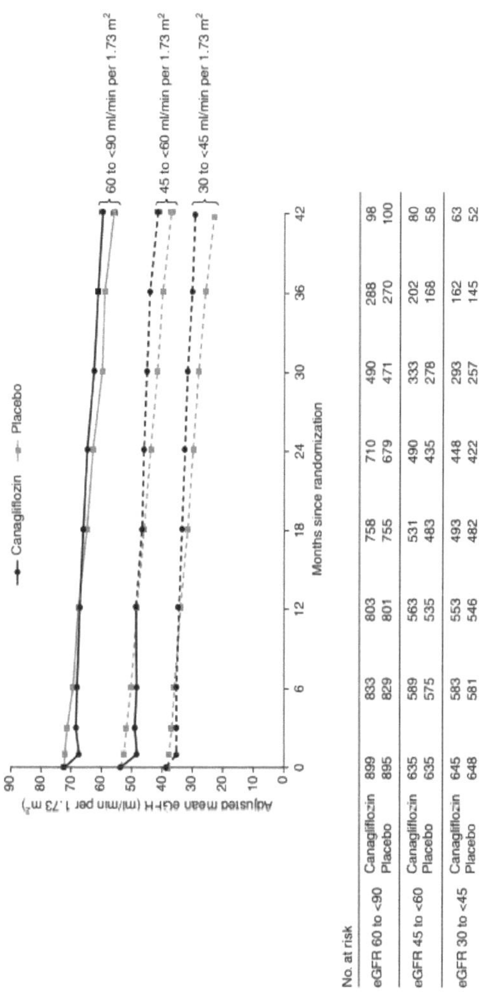

Figure 13: **Effect of canagliflozin on eGFR** (CREDENCE), Meg J. Jardine et al. (136).

Canagliflozin caused an acute fall in eGFR that was mildest in those with an eGFR of 30-45 ml/min per 1.73 m2 at screening, followed by a slower decline in eGFR in each eGFR category at screening. The slope lines cross at the corresponding point at 14.3, 11.2 and 8.7 months for those whose initial eGFR was between 60 and 90, 45 and 60, and 30 and 45 ml/min per 1.73 m2, respectively. On-treatment eGFR On-treatment eGFR includes all central laboratory measurements of eGFR from day 1 of the study to the last dose plus 2 days. Changes in eGFR from baseline were analyzed using a restricted maximum likelihood repeated measures approach.

Subsequently, patients randomized to placebo experienced an eGFR decline of 4.59 ml/min per 1.73 m^2 per year, with similar declines in all eGFR categories. Canagliflozin caused a slower decline in eGFR in all eGFR categories compared with placebo (all P<0.001), and there was no evidence of a difference in benefit between eGFR subgroups (P heterogeneity =0.65). Canagliflozin improved overall slope, the combined effect of acute effects and chronic change in slope between baseline and week 130, overall and in all eGFR subgroups (all P<0.001), with no evidence of differences between eGFR subgroups (P heterogeneity =0.71).

In patients with an eGFR between 30 and 45 ml/min per 1.73 m^2 (the group closest to the threshold for dialysis initiation), canagliflozin produced a significant decrease in eGFR of 2.03 (95% CI, 1.34 to 2.73) ml/min per 1.73 m^2 , there was a subsequent reduction in eGFR of 2,61 (95% CI 2.06 to 3.16) ml/min per 1.73 m^2 per year compared with patients receiving placebo (mean [SD] decrease of 1.85 [0.13] in patients receiving canagliflozin vs. 4.59 [0.14] in patients receiving placebo).

2.5. The absolute effect of canagliflozin

While the relative benefit of canagliflozin versus placebo was generally consistent across all eGFR subgroups, for all renal outcomes except dialysis, transplantation or renal death, absolute benefits were greatest in the lowest eGFR subgroups (all heterogeneities P <0.03), where effects were consistent between subgroups (P heterogeneity =0.06; Figure 10). There were no significant differences in absolute benefit for cardiovascular events between eGFR subgroups, with the exception of the composite endpoint of cardiovascular death or hospitalized heart failure, where there was borderline evidence that absolute benefits were greater in the lower eGFR subgroups (P heterogeneity=0.096; Figure 11).

2.6. Impact on intermediate results

In participants in the eGFR screening subgroups, canagliflozin reduced HbA1c, blood pressure, body weight and proteinuria compared with placebo. Compared with placebo, canagliflozin had a lower hypoglycemic effect and a greater reduction in blood pressure in participants with lower baseline eGFR, while reductions in body weight and proteinuria were similar in all subgroups.

2.7. Experience of people whose last treatment eGFR <30 ml/min per 1.73 m^2.

In the CREDENCE study, a large number of participants had an eGFR < 30 ml/min per 1.73 m^2. For the subgroup of participants who completed treatment with an eGFR < 30 ml/min per 1.73 m^2 (n = 929; canagliflozin, n = 417; placebo, n = 512), mean follow-up to the first eGFR < 30 ml/min per 1.73 m^2 was 12.9 months (canagliflozin, 11.7 months; placebo, 13.8 months), while mean follow-up thereafter was 19.3 months (canagliflozin, 20.5 months; placebo, 18.4 months). The relative number of events following an initial reduction in eGFR to < 30 ml/min per 1.73 m^2 in the canagliflozin and placebo groups was similar to that in the overall trial. Because these analyses were based on comparisons of post-randomization events (eGFR down to <30 ml/min per 1.73 m^2), they are not randomized and should be considered exploratory, but may help to illustrate the evolution of participants throughout the study.

3. Discussion

Canagliflozin consistently and reliably prevented renal and cardiovascular events in significantly albuminuric participants with eGFR categories of 30-45, 45-60 and 60-90 ml/min per 1.73 m^2. These benefits were achieved in the context of the widespread use of renin-angiotensin system inhibitors. Although relative benefits were consistent across all eGFR categories, increasing rates of renal and cardiovascular events were observed as eGFR levels decreased, while absolute benefits were greater in lower eGFR subgroups. The beneficial effect of canagliflozin on the occurrence of clinical events was reinforced by the observed reduction in the rate of chronic decline in renal function, which was reduced by >50% in all three subgroups. Specifically, canagliflozin attenuated chronic eGFR decline by 60% and 65% in patients with baseline eGFR of 30-45 ml/min per 1.73 m^2 and 45-60 ml/min per 1.73 m^2, respectively.
Reassuringly, participants with eGFR between 30 and 45 ml/min per 1.73 m^2 did not experience excessive major safety issues, and observational analysis did not show that when eGFR fell to 30 ml/min per 1.73 m^2, benefits varied. Overall, these results support the initiation of canagliflozin in patients with eGFR between 30 and 90 ml/min/1.73 m^2 and significant albuminuria, and the continuation of treatment below this threshold. Treatment below this threshold.

The effect of canagliflozin versus placebo on intermediate outcomes was broadly consistent with that observed in previous studies. As expected, the hypoglycemic effect of canagliflozin was attenuated in patients with deteriorating renal function. However, reductions in albuminuria, body weight and blood pressure were generally similar in the eGFR subgroups. The sharp initial fall in eGFR observed in the CREDENCE study was an established response to initiation of treatment with canagliflozin (134)and the subsequent attenuation of the eGFR decline was consistent with a reduction in intraglomerular pressure, which may have helped protect the kidneys (137-139). Other potential mechanisms of renal protection are being actively investigated (140-142). The data strongly suggest that CREDENCE has a glucose-independent mechanism of renal and cardiovascular benefit.

Although uncertainty remains as to the relative importance of several underlying mechanisms, CREDENCE identified clear benefits on renal clinical outcomes (132). This important new finding demonstrates that renal and cardiac protection is preserved in patients who started treatment with an eGFR between 30 and 45 ml/min per 1.73 m^2, providing further insight into the underlying mechanism of action. Despite the reduced effect on glycemic control, the clinical benefit proved significant, raising the important question of whether these drugs would benefit kidney disease in a non-diabetic setting. Ongoing trials enrolling patients with non-diabetic kidney disease should provide important additional information (NCT03036150, NCT03594110, NCT03190694).

Similarly, three large cardiovascular outcome trials have demonstrated the benefit of SGLT2 inhibitors in preventing hospitalization for heart failure in participants with largely preserved renal function (120,121) although the exact mechanism of heart failure attenuation is uncertain. These drugs have natriuretic effects, which can lead to early reductions in blood pressure and weight, and may contribute to the early benefit of hospitalization for heart failure. However, despite a stable volume, benefits continued to accrue over time. The CREDENCE study confirmed that people with lower eGFR and higher risk of heart failure had a greater absolute benefit from hospitalization for heart failure. An important aspect of the CREDENCE study in the SGLT2 inhibitor trial was the intention to continue treatment even if eGFR fell below 30 ml/min per 1.73 m^2. We provide observational reports of events occurring once eGFR fell to <30 ml/min/1.73 m^2 in patients whose eGFR remained <30 ml/min/1.73 m^2 at the end of treatment, in analyses that are limited by their dependence on an outcome that occurs well after randomization. The ongoing DIAMOND (NCT03190694) and DAPA-CKD (NCT03036150) trials are recruiting participants with an eGFR of less than 25 ml/min per 1.73 m^2, while the EMPA-KIDNEY (NCT03594110) trial included patients with an eGFR of less than 20 ml/min per 1.73 m^2. Taken together, these trials will provide evidence of the effect of SGLT2 inhibitors in patients with low eGFR at treatment initiation. At the same time, the overall concordance between our exploratory report and the results of the CREDENCE study reassures us that there is no reason to refuse continued treatment with CREDENCE until chronic dialysis is initiated or a kidney transplant is performed.

The CREDENCE study was designed to examine the prognostic impact of canagliflozin in people at risk of progression of diabetic kidney disease. It therefore has the advantage of including a population with significant proteinuria (high risk of renal and cardiovascular events) and randomization stratified by eGFR category so that most participants had an eGFR < 60 ml/min/1.73 m^2, providing a robust estimate of canagliflozin for a population with an eGFR reduced to 30 ml/min per 1.73 m^2.

In addition, careful evaluation of renal events by central eGFR assessment requires chronic outcomes to be documented as sustained and adjudication of renal and other important events. Results may not be generalizable to patients who started treatment with an eGFR <30 ml/min/1.73 m^2. Again, the results also apply to people with severe albuminuria, although the results are consistent with those of the CANVAS project (most participants had little or no albuminuria). The trial was stopped prematurely due to significant efficacy on the primary endpoint, which may have limited the ability to assess the impact of secondary and safety endpoints. Analyses of participants who completed treatment at eGFR <30 ml/min/1.73 m^2 were reported by the randomized group, however, since the cohort was defined by post-randomization events, they would be confounded and subject to bias, Including survival bias and conflict bias, and should only be considered as hypothesis-generating data.

Canagliflozin was safe in preventing clinically important renal and cardiovascular events in patients with diabetes mellitus, macroalbuminuria and eGFR between 30 and 90 ml/min per 1.73 m^2 at baseline. These effects appeared to be consistent across all eGFR categories, with lower eGFR categories showing greater absolute benefits on renal parameters. They support extending the initiation of canagliflozin therapy to patients with an eGFR of 30 to <45 ml/min/1.73 m^2, and generally continuing treatment until initiation of dialysis, or renal transplantation.

IX. Place of SGLT2 inhibitors in acute heart failure

Acute heart failure (AHF) is a major public health problem, affecting nearly 6 million people in the United States and 26 million worldwide (143). AHF is defined as the onset or rapid worsening of signs and symptoms of heart failure (HF) that require urgent medical attention (144). With over one million hospitalizations annually in the U.S., AHF is the leading cause of hospitalization in the elderly (143). Approximately 3 out of 1 patients with FHA are readmitted within 5 days of discharge, and more than 30 out of 3 are readmitted within the first year (145). Mortality rates at 4 years range from 1 to 10%, with the highest risk of mortality within 30 days of index hospitalization (145-147). Despite therapeutic advances in the treatment of chronic heart failure (CHF) (148)AHF has a poor prognosis, since no treatment has been shown to have a long-term benefit on mortality (149). Loop diuretics are the mainstay of AHF treatment, but have a negative impact on renal function as well as a potential neurohormonal imbalance (150-152).

A metanalysis by Noor Ul Amin et al. assessed the efficacy of SGLT2 inhibitors versus placebo for primary endpoints, including all-cause and cardiovascular mortality, heart failure events, symptom improvement and readmissions. The secondary endpoint was the risk of serious adverse events. Only randomized controlled trials (RCTs) involving adult patients (>18 years) hospitalized with de novo AHF, acute decompensated chronic heart failure with reduced, borderline or preserved ejection, and receiving SGLT2 inhibitors were included. A quantitative analysis methodology was applied where standardized mean difference (SMD) applying 95% confidence intervals (CI) for continuous outcomes and hazard ratio (HR) with 95% CI was obtained. All tests were performed on Review Manager 5.4 (Cochrane). A total of three RCTs were included in a total of 1,831 patients, 49.9% of whom received SGLT2 inhibitors. The mean age was 72.9 years in the intervention group, versus 70.6 years in the placebo group. Only 33.7% of the sample were women. Follow-up ranged from 2 to 9 months. Heart failure events were reduced by 62% in the intervention group (RR = 0.66, p < 0.0001). Readmissions were reduced by 24% with SGLT2 inhibitors (RR = 0.76, p = 0.03). The efficacy and safety of SGLT2 inhibitors in preventing post-AHF complications were also evaluated. Rates of all-cause mortality, cardiovascular mortality, heart failure and readmissions were significantly reduced during the first 1-9 months of hospitalization.

SGLT2 inhibitors were found to reduce the risk of all-cause mortality by 27%, and were significant at 51% when post-sensitivity analysis was performed. In addition, we also found a significant 28% reduction in cardiovascular mortality and heart failure events in patients receiving SGLT2 inhibitors. In addition, we found a significant 24% reduction in first readmission rates in patients on SGLT2 inhibitors. These results were supported by significant symptomatic improvement and no additional safety concerns. (153).

The first evidence of the efficacy of SGLT2 inhibitors in clinical trials was seen in the EMPA-REG-OUTCOME (154)where it was noted that people hospitalized for heart failure and randomized to treatment groups had a twofold reduced risk of rehospitalization or death within the first 1-3 months after the first heart failure event (154). The EMPA-RESPONSE-AHF trial was the first prospective clinical trial to assess the clinical benefits of SGLT2 inhibitors in patients with acute heart failure (155). It was a double-blind study, randomizing patients between placebo and parallel groups, in several centers; 80 people with acute heart failure with or without type 2 diabetes mellitus were randomized to receive 10 mg / day empagliflozin or in the control group with monitoring within 24 hours of admission (155). The EMPULSE trial (EMPagliflozin in hospitalized patients with acUte heart infection who have been stabilized) was based in several centers, randomized in a double-blind setting where the effects of the

SGLT2 inhibitor (empagliflozin) were evaluated for safety, clinical benefit and tolerability in acute heart failure (156,157). In this trial, patients underwent an initial stabilization period lasting a median of 3 days. Patients also received 10 mg daily of the SGLT2 inhibitor (empagliflozin) or no intervention with standard care for 90 days.

The EMPULSE trial met its endpoint, where patients showed more clinical benefit compared with placebo; the stratified benefit ratio was 1.36 (95% CI = 1.09 to 1.68, p = 0.0054) (156). Notably, the benefits were unanimous across different subgroups, including those with chronic decompensated heart failure and ventricular ejection fractions up or down by 40%. The intervention was considered both well tolerated and safe for patients.

Other representatives of the class, including dapagliflozin, are currently under investigation. DISTATE-AHF, a multicenter, prospective, open-label, randomized trial enrolling 240 patients in the USA (147). The patient population consists of patients with type 2 diabetes mellitus hospitalized with acute hypervolemic heart failure and a glomerular filtration rate greater than 30 mL/min/1.73 m2 (With endpoints including diuretic response, inpatient AHF, 30-day readmission rate and safety parameters, it remains to be quantified whether dapagliflozin will be a candidate treatment for AHF in diabetic patients) (147). In the CHIEF-HF trial, 30 participants with heart failure, regardless of diabetes or ejection fraction status, were randomized to receive canagliflozin (467 mg) or a placebo intervention (100 mg). Although enrollment was stopped prematurely due to sponsor priorities, Spertus and colleagues in 2022 report that the primary endpoint of the KCCQ TBS was changed at 12 weeks by 4.3 points (p = 0.016) in favor of canagliflozin (158). CHIEF-HF met its primary endpoint, with a paradigm shift in the management of acute heart failure, although it is important to further test and examine the results of SGLT2 inhibitors in randomized, double-blind settings.

Thus, the three RCTs published in this field to date were analyzed. The EMPULSE trial functions as an addition/complement to the results of the two previous trials that administered SGLT2 inhibitors; these trials describe the patient journey from acute heart failure to hospital admission and treatment use (159). The results confirm that SGLT2 inhibitors help manage patients with acute heart failure after hospitalization.

Finally, the limitations of this meta-analysis should be noted. Firstly, the duration of intervention varied from trial to trial. Secondly, there was little consistency in the way trials defined heart failure events. Third, the duration of follow-up was not uniform. Some aspects of care were administered for longer periods during the trials. Fourth, outcome measures were taken at different times, for example readmission rates. Fifth, the sample size was quite small, with participants enrolled in the SGLT2 inhibitor group not achieving generalizability. Finally, the majority of the sample was diabetic, which may lead to biases in decision-making.

X. Efficacy and safety of SGLT-2 inhibitors for the treatment of diabetes mellitus in renal transplant recipients

An initial meta-analysis (160) demonstrates the efficacy and safety of inhibitors

SGLT-2 inhibitors in diabetic kidney transplant patients. Treatment with SGLT-2 inhibitors was effective in lowering HbA1C and inducing weight loss, when taken for at least 12 months and 6 months respectively. Furthermore, eGFR, serum creatinine levels and urinary protein/creatinine ratios remained stable throughout follow-up in patients receiving SGLT-2 inhibitors. Empagliflozin was effective in reducing weight, and canagliflozin was effective in reducing HbA1C and blood pressure. Adverse effects of SGLT-2 inhibitors included urinary tract infection (43.8%), small lower-limb ulcers (10%), cellulitis (10%), acute renal failure (3.6%) and genital mycosis (1.4%). No cases of normoglycemic ketoacidosis or acute rejection were reported.

SGLT-2 inhibitors inhibit sodium and glucose reabsorption in the proximal renal tubule, causing osmotic diuresis and natriuresis (161). As a result, glucose and HbA1C levels decrease (161,162). However, this glycemic efficacy is modest and limited by filtered glucose loading and osmotic diuresis (163,164). A recent meta-analysis of SGLT-2 inhibitors in non-renal transplanted diabetic patients with chronic renal failure showed improved efficacy of SGLT-2. HbA1C, body weight and proteinuria (165) were slightly lower in non-transplanted diabetic patients with chronic renal failure.

In this study, the results in kidney transplant recipients (160) suggest a similar effect, with the exception of albuminuria. The effect of reducing HbA1C by around 0.6% in diabetic kidney transplant recipients (160) is consistent with previously reported mean reductions of 0.4% to 1.1% in general diabetic patients (163,164). With regard to body weight, previous literature has reported a weight loss of 2 to 3 kg in renal transplant patients with diabetes. Diabetic patients treated with SGLT-2 inhibitors lost 2 to 3 kg of body weight (163,166). This result is consistent with the weight loss of 2 kg (160). These results show that SGLT-2 inhibitors are effective in kidney transplant recipients with diabetes and in non-transplant diabetic populations (163,166).

With regard to preservation of renal function, this study (160) showed no significant changes in eGFR, serum creatinine or urinary protein. Although the follow-up period (6 to 12 months) may not have been long enough to observe these differences, at least during these follow-up periods, there was no deterioration in renal function in diabetic kidney transplant recipients treated with ISGLT-2. Previous large clinical trials with empagliflozin (EMPA-REG OUTCOME) and canagliflozin (CANVAS Program) have suggested an advantage of SGLT-2 inhibitors in reducing the progression of proteinuria (16) (167). However, due to limited data, there was no control group and it could not be concluded that treatment with SGLT-2 inhibitors helps to slow the progression of proteinuria in diabetic kidney transplant recipients (160).

With regard to blood pressure, weight loss, combined with osmotic diuresis and reduction in total body sodium, could theoretically lead to a 4-6 mm Hg reduction in systolic blood pressure PAS and a 1-2 mm Hg reduction in diastolic blood pressure PAD, as demonstrated in non-renal transplant patients with diabetes (168). However, this study (160) showed no significant reduction in blood pressure in renal transplant patients treated with SGLT-2 inhibitors. This could be explained by more complex pathogenic mechanisms of hypertension in kidney transplant recipients, including, but not limited to, side effects of immunosuppressive therapy and the presence of native kidneys (169,170). Another possible explanation is that the sample size was insufficient to detect these differences (160). Although we observed a reduction in systolic blood pressure in patients treated with canagliflozin, but not in patients treated with empagliflozin (160)these discordant effects may be due to different baseline characteristics, such as higher eGFR and shorter transplant duration, which may reflect better graft function with canagliflozin compared with empagliflozin.

In addition to reducing glomerular hyperfiltration and hypertension, SGLT-2 inhibitors are anti-inflammatory, anti-fibrotic and protective against extracellular matrix deregulation by reducing tumor necrosis factor (TNF 1) receptor, interleukin 6 (IL -6), matrix metalloproteinase 7 and fibronectin 1 (171). In addition, SGLT-2 inhibitors also reduce serum levels of leptin, C-reactive protein and interleukin 1β (IL-1β) secretion via the Reactive oxygen species of NOD Like Receptor pyrin 3 caspase 1 (ROS-NLRP3-caspase-1) pathway (172,173). In addition, SGLT-2 inhibitors also exhibit antioxidant effects via activation of SIRT1/AMPK and inhibition of the protein kinase B/mTOR (Akt/mTOR) signaling pathway (174). Some studies have also found a reduction in myeloperoxidase levels in the SGLT-2 inhibitor group, suggesting a reduction in oxidative damage to the vascular endothelium (175). These potential effects of SGLT-2 inhibitors may be beneficial for kidney transplant recipients, as inflammation and fibrosis are the main causes of allograft rejection.

Given the safety of SGLT-2 inhibitors in diabetic kidney transplant recipients, the incidence of urinary tract infections in this study (160) was 43.8%, while the incidence of urinary tract infections in general renal transplant recipients was 38.0%. (176). No significant difference between the two ($p = 0.13$). These findings were confirmed by a previous meta-analysis of the non-transplant diabetic population, which found an increased risk of genital infections but not urinary tract infections (177). In this study (160)we found 1.4% genital mycoses. However, due to lack of data, we did not have a control group or a reported incidence in kidney transplant recipients in general to make comparisons. SGLT-2 inhibitors have been associated with a higher risk of euglycemic ketoacidosis via a mechanism involving decreased insulin and increased glucagon secretion, thus stimulating the switch from glucose to fat metabolism and promoting ketogenesis (178) (179).

However, the studies included in this meta-analysis (160) reported no cases of normoglycemic ketoacidosis. However, sample size or duration of follow-up may not have been sufficient to detect this event. In non-renal transplant patients, a slight increase in serum creatinine has been observed during the first 3-6 weeks of treatment with an SGLT-2 inhibitor, accompanied by an early decrease in eGFR (approx. 4 ml/min/1.73 m^2), and the data confirm this (162) (180). The decrease in serum creatinine and increase in eGFR after discontinuation of SGLT-2 inhibitors suggest the functional nature of the reduction in GFR induced by these drugs (162,180). However, a case of biopsy-confirmed nephropathy in a non-renal transplant diabetic patient receiving canagliflozin has recently been reported (181).

Subgroup analyses investigated the effect of SGLT-2 inhibitors according to the type of SGLT-2 inhibitor and the change in each parameter at 6 and 12 months (160).

XI. Adverse reactions and safety

Although the safety profile is favourable, there are some notable side effects of iSGLT2 :

- Mycotic urogenital infections such as balanitis in men and vulvovaginitis in women (182)These are generally benign and easily curable, although rare cases of Fournier's gangrene have been reported. The negative effect of SGLT2 inhibitors on the incidence of genital tract infections has been extensively studied. The FDA also recently issued a safety advisory concerning the use of SGLT2 inhibitors after 12 cases of Fournier's gangrene were reported (183). A meta-analysis of 12 randomized, placebo-controlled phase 2b/3 trials revealed that dapagliflozin significantly increased the risk of vulvovaginitis and balanitis infections (184). Another double-blind, placebo-controlled study reported a higher incidence of genital infections in people using dapagliflozin (185). Infections in these studies were mostly mild to moderate, responded to standard treatments and generally did not require discontinuation of the SGLT2 inhibitor. Data compiled on canagliflozin use and genital tract infections indicate a high incidence of infections at the start of SGLT2 inhibitor therapy (first 24-26 weeks), but the frequency of infections decreased significantly over time (186).

- Dehydration and hypovolemia through osmotic diuresis associated with natriuresis, iSGLT2 can theoretically lead to a risk of dehydration with arterial hypotension, particularly orthostatic hypotension. (187) ;
- Hypoglycemia: The risk of hypoglycemia is increased when SGLT2 is administered concomitantly with insulin secretagogues such as sulfonamides or insulin. Physicians should reduce the dose of insulin secretagogue or insulin when combined with SGLT2 inhibitors. One study indicates that the risk of hypoglycemia is higher in elderly patients taking SGLT2 inhibitors. (188).
- Normoglycemic ketoacidosis: diabetic ketoacidosis (DKA) is strongly associated with type 1 diabetes, but euglycemic DKA is also observed in type 2 diabetics with severe disease or predisposition to ketosis. There are three potential mechanisms of DKA in type 2 diabetics: insulinopenia, the creation of counter-regulatory stress hormones and elevated free fatty acids. SGLT2 inhibitors lower the insulin/glucagon ratio and increase lipolysis, which stimulates the production of ketone bodies in the liver (189). A recent study on diabetic rats treated with SGLT2 inhibitors suggested that insulinopenia and dehydration are key factors in the development of ketoacidosis (190). Cases of euglycemic DKA have been reported in the literature in patients with type 2 diabetes on SGLT2 inhibitors (191,192). However, multiple meta-analyses have revealed no

increased risk of DKA in patients taking SGLT2 inhibitors versus placebo (193,194).

Normoglycemic ketoacidosis, reported in EMPA-REG OUTCOME and CANVAS, and a significant excess risk in DECLARE-TIMI 58, with an atypical presentation known as euglycemia, explained by the mechanism of action of this therapy (increased glucagon levels, hypovolemia, reduced urinary excretion of ketone bodies...).The prescribing physician should discuss with the patient the manifestations and management of this complication. (195) ;

- Lower-limb amputations and non-vertebral fractures reported only for Canagliflozin, while the underlying mechanisms are not yet well elucidated (182,196).

In the CANVAS study, canagliflozin showed a risk of distal amputation with a relative risk of around 2 (121) . In 2017, the FDA reported an elevated amputation risk, it is greater for iSGLT2, particularly for Canagliflozin (197). But in January 2020, the FDA cancelled the Precautions for Use for canagliflozin and the risk of distal amputations (http://www.fda.gov/drugs/drug-safety-andavailability/fda-removes-boxed-warning-about-risk-leg-andfoot-amputations-diabetes-medicine-canagliflozin). The FDA certainly reminds all prescribers of the need to monitor diabetic feet, whether treated with iSGLT2 or not, especially in patients considered to have chronic renal failure, in whom, There is a risk of distal arterial damage.

Amputations were mainly in the toe or metatarsal, and the risk compared with placebo remained constant in people with peripheral vascular disease and a history of amputations (196). The increased risk of amputation with canagliflozin was similar when calculated using both the difference in restricted mean survival time (RMST) and hazard ratio (HR) (198). Empagliflozin was not associated with a risk of lower-limb amputation (199).

A retrospective cohort study of 953,906 diabetic patients found an association between the initiation of treatment with SGLT2 inhibitors and an increased risk of amputation compared with metformin, sulfonylureas and thiazolidinediones. However, this difference was not significant when SGLT2 inhibitors were compared with DPP-4 inhibitors or GLP-1 agonists (200).

As for the risk of bone fractures: type 2 diabetic patients experience paradoxical bone effects as a result of their disease. Numerous studies and meta-analyses confirm that patients with type 2 diabetes have higher bone mineral density on DEXA scans, but are much more likely to suffer hip fractures (201-203).

The consequences of SGLT2 inhibitors on this paradoxical effect of diabetes are unclear and controversial. Animal studies show that canagliflozin adversely affects bone microarchitecture, bone strength and bone mineral density (204,205). Similarly, a clinical trial with canagliflozin observed a reduction in bone mineral density at the hip, but not at other bone sites on DEXA scintigraphy. There is evidence that reduced bone mineral density may be related to weight loss and decreased estradiol (206). Kohan et al described fractures with dapagliflozin administration, but the location of the fractures was more indicative of falls than bone density problems (207). In the Canagliflozin Cardiovascular Assessment Study (CANVAS), the incidence of fractures compared with placebo was statistically significantly higher (4.0% vs. 2.6%). However, further analysis of the CANVAS data revealed that statistical significance no longer existed after excluding fractures not associated with osteoporosis or skeletal fragility (208). In contrast, multiple meta-analyses conclude that SGLT2 inhibitors are not associated with an increased risk of fractures. These analyses include 58 peer-reviewed studies and a total of 38,670 patients (209).

On the other hand, patients and their physicians will be happy to reduce usual weight by 2 to 3 kg and systolic blood pressure by 4 mm Hg, and above all that there is no hypoglycemia associated directly with the use of iSGLT2 (168).

- Cancer risk: The link between SGLT2 inhibitors and cancer has been extensively studied and remains controversial today. When dapagliflozin was submitted for FDA approval, it was denied in 2011 due to concerns about increased risk of bladder and breast cancer. Pooled studies of dapagliflozin showed that 9 of 5478 patients on dapagliflozin versus 1 of 3156 control patients developed bladder and breast cancer (210). A first meta-analysis evaluating the safety of SGLT2 inhibitors also found an imbalance in the incidence of bladder and breast cancers compared with control subjects (211). In order to obtain FDA approval, the recently published DECLARE-TIMI 58 trial, which evaluated over 17,000 patients, was created to assess the long-term effects of dapagliflozin. The study found that dapagliflozin was associated with a lower rate of bladder cancer than placebo, and that there was no difference in breast cancer compared with placebo (212).

A recent meta-analysis by Tang et al highlighted a statistically significant increase in the risk of bladder cancer, particularly with empagliflozin (OR 3.87 [95% CI 1.48, 10.09]). Canagliflozin was associated with a statistically significant reduction in the incidence of gastrointestinal cancer (213). However, the data used in this analysis have been disputed. Four cases of bladder cancer were not included in the analysis, nor was causality assessed at patient level. With the corrected data, the association between bladder cancer and SGLT2 inhibitors became non-statistically significant. (214). Another recent meta-analysis of 27 clinical trials found no statistically significant increase in the risk of any type of cancer with SGLT2 (215).

- Lipids: SGLT2 inhibitors may cause a slight dose-dependent increase in HDL and LDL cholesterol levels. Numerous studies, including the EMPA-REG OUTCOME trial, have associated empagliflozin with increases in HDL-C and LDL-C compared with placebo (216-219). A meta-analysis of SGLT2 inhibitor trials reported an increase in HDL-C and LDL-C and a decrease in triglycerides compared with placebo (220). Studies of canagliflozin, including the CANVAS trial, also reported similar increases in HDL and LDL cholesterol (186,196). Another study showed that dapagliflozin increased both LDL and HDL cholesterol. However, there was a decrease in atherogenic low-density LDL cholesterol and an increase in less atherogenic high-density LDL cholesterol (221).

The mechanism by which SGLT2 inhibitors alter lipids is not fully understood, but is probably a combination of hemoconcentration and reduced LDL receptor activity in the liver. Reduced hepatic LDL receptor expression is probably due to increased HMG-CoA reductase activity (222,223).

- Electrolyte imbalance: multiple meta-analyses have shown that SGLT2 inhibitors cause a small percentage of changes in serum electrolyte levels. Canagliflozin was associated with a statistically significant increase in serum magnesium levels, which operated in a dose-dependent manner. Empagliflozin and dapagliflozin also produced a statistically significant increase in magnesium levels. However, dapagliflozin increased serum magnesium levels only at a dose of 10 mg. With regard to sodium levels, a difference was observed between empagliflozin and canagliflozin. The 25 mg empagliflozin dose increased serum sodium levels, while the 300 mg canagliflozin dose decreased them. SGLT2 inhibitors slightly increase serum phosphate levels. Analyses showed that potassium and calcium levels were unaffected by SGLT2 inhibitors. (224-226).

It is possible that increased magnesium and phosphate levels are partly responsible for the reduction in cardiovascular events seen in the EMPA-REG OUTCOME study thanks to the prevention of arrhythmias (218). However, increased phosphate may also be responsible for the negative side effects on bone density and fractures seen with SGLT2 inhibitors in the CANVAS study. Increased phosphate leads to higher levels of parathyroid hormone, which accelerates bone resorption. Increased fibroblast growth factor 23 (FGF-23) levels are also associated with increased phosphate levels, leading to a decrease in serum vitamin D concentration (227).

- Drug interactions and interference between drugs and laboratory tests :

- The risk of hypoglycemia increases when SGLT2 inhibitors are combined with an insulin secretagogue (e.g. sulfonamide) or insulin. Therefore, clinicians should reduce the dose of insulin/insulin secretagogue to reduce the risk of hypoglycemia (188).
  SGLT2 inhibitors, including empagliflozin, decrease sodium-glucose and lithium-glucose reabsorption in the proximal connecting tubules, thereby increasing renal excretion of sodium, glucose and lithium. Concomitant use of an SGLT2 inhibitor and lithium may reduce serum lithium concentrations (228).
- Canagliflozin increases the maximum plasma concentration (Cmax:36%) and the area under the curve (AUC:20%) of digoxin. Given the narrow therapeutic index of digoxin, therapeutic monitoring of digoxin is recommended. (229).
- UGT enzyme inducers, such as rifampicin, phenytoin, ritonavir and phenobarbital, reduce canagliflozin exposure (AUC), which may reduce canagliflozin efficacy. Consider increasing the dose of canagliflozin when used with UGT (230).

- False-positive urine glucose test: The sodium-glucose cotransporter SGLT2 in the proximal tubule is the pathway for renal glucose reabsorption. Inhibition of SGLT2 increases urinary glucose. Monitoring of glycemic control in patients taking SGLT2 inhibitors by means of urinalysis is not recommended in diabetic patients (231).
- The structure of 1,5-Anhydroglucitol (1,5-AG) is similar to that of glucose. Monitoring of glycemic control by 1,5-AG assay is not reliable for assessing glycemic control in patients taking SGLT2 (232).
- Non-selective beta-blockers can mask the symptoms of hypoglycemia, and SGLT2 inhibitors are known to induce hypoglycemia; thus, concomitant administration of beta-blockers and SGLT2 inhibitors requires caution (233).

The classic contraindication is an eGFR of less than 45 or 60 ml/min/1.73 m^2, depending on the molecule, due to loss of efficacy and not for safety reasons; studies carried out to date have shown an increased risk of genital infections, whereas the occurrence of the other adverse effects listed above was negligible. A history of urogenital infection or lower-limb arteriopathy should therefore preclude their prescription.

XII. Toxicity

There is no antidote for SGLT-2 inhibitors, nor are they eliminated by dialysis. A retrospective study of SGLT2 inhibitor overdoses reported to 13 U.S. poison control centers revealed that most cases of mild exposure did not develop hypoglycemia, with the exception of children. Instead, they experienced nausea, vomiting or dizziness. However, intentional overdosage of SGLT2 inhibitors can lead to hypoglycemia, vomiting, confusion, hypertension, tachycardia and urinary incontinence (234). One case report describes euglycemia despite an overdose of ertugliflozin. The patient had accidentally ingested 150 mg ertugliflozin, whereas the maximum recommended dose is 15 mg (235).

According to standard hypoglycemia protocol, treatment requires immediate correction of hypoglycemia with oral glucose if the patient can eat - for patients with impaired consciousness, dextrose (25 g) is administered IV to treat hypoglycemia. If no IV access has been established, glucagon (0.5 to 1 mg SC/IM) is administered immediately. In case of refractory hypoglycemia, subcutaneous/intravenous octreotide has been used. In case of complicated overdose, contact the Poison Control Center (235).

XIII. New applications

1. **Non-alcoholic hepatic steatosis**: non-alcoholic hepatic steatosis is defined as an accumulation of fat in the liver associated with insulin resistance and the presence of steatosis in >5% of hepatocytes on histological analysis. This includes hepatic steatosis caused by non-alcoholic steatohepatitis (NASH), cirrhosis or simple steatosis. NAFLD does not include diseases due to excessive alcohol consumption, hepatitis, drugs or other rare conditions (236). Type 2 diabetes and insulin resistance are strongly associated with NAFLD. The prevalence of NAFLD in type 2 diabetes is estimated at 69% to 87%, depending on the imaging modality used, compared with 30% in the general population (237). Patients with NAFLD are at increased risk of cirrhosis and hepatocellular carcinoma (238).

A reduction in serum alanine aminotransferase (ALAT) of 30% or more from baseline was predictive of improved liver fibrosis progression in patients with NASH (239). A pilot study by Seko et al examined the use of 100 mg canagliflozin for 12 weeks in type 2 diabetic patients with NASH at various stages. They found that canagliflozin reduced ALAT by an average of 23.9 U/L, and that the greatest benefit was seen in patients with early-stage NASH versus those with more advanced fibrosis. The authors also encouraged a larger, more robust study to confirm their findings, as the sample size was small (240). Animal studies have shed light on the mechanism behind the protective effects of SGLT2 inhibitors on NASH. Canagliflozin was shown to increase zinc-α2-glycoprotein (ZAG) levels, reduce hepatic inflammatory cytokines and increase Bcl-2 expression. It also reduced oxidative stress in the liver and enhanced antioxidant capacity (241).

2. **Weight loss/obesity:** SGLT2 inhibitors induce dose-dependent weight loss. Meta-analyses estimate a weight loss effect of

around 1.5 to 2.5 kg (242). However, these weight-loss effects are slowed by an increase in energy intake (243). Another study reported that 150 mg licogliflozin, a Japanese dual inhibitor of SGLT1/SGLT2, significantly reduced the body weight of obese non-diabetic individuals by 5.7% compared with placebo. A positive effect on incretin hormones was also observed (244). Numerous clinical trials are currently investigating the usefulness of SGLT2 inhibitors in non-diabetic obese individuals. Although probably not effective enough as a monotherapy for obesity, SGLT2 inhibitors could potentially be effective for weight loss when combined with other drugs that reduce food intake.

3. **Early-stage lung adenocarcinoma**

A recent study implicated SGLT2 expression in the early development of lung tumors, both in precancerous lung lesions and in early-stage adenocarcinoma. Scafoglio et al found that selective targeting of SGLT2 by canagliflozin significantly prolonged survival rates in mice (245). However, the effect was not permanent, as tumor growth eventually escaped SGLT2 inhibition, probably due to up regulation of SGLT2. The researchers were also able to modify proton emission tomography (PET) to track SGLT2 activity, which could prove useful in assessing the response of early-stage lung lesions to SGLT2 inhibitor treatment. Further studies testing the use of SGLT2 inhibitors in early-stage lung adenocarcinoma are required before the clinical significance of these findings can be determined (245).

4. **Cardiovascular fitness:** increasing physical activity is one of the key lifestyle changes recommended for the treatment of type 2 diabetes. Diabetic patients show a decrease in cardiovascular fitness, skeletal muscle mass and overall physical activity levels (246,247). Numerous studies have demonstrated that glitazones and glucagon-like peptide-1 (GLP-1) agonists have positive

effects on cardiovascular capacity (248-250). Two pilot studies were set up to determine whether empagliflozin improved levels of cardiovascular capacity in patients with type 2 diabetes and congestive heart failure. In patients taking loop diuretics, both studies revealed a significant improvement in VO2max. In contrast, patients not taking loop diuretics did not enjoy the same benefits. It is hypothesized that the synergistic effect of the two drugs is due to the increased sodium supply to the distal tubules, which amplifies the natriuretic effect of the diuretics (251,252).

XIV. Future SGLT2 inhibitors

Sotagliflozin (LX4211) is unique in that it has a dual inhibitory effect on SGLT1/SGLT2. Compared with canagliflozin and dapagliflozin, sotagliflozin has a similar inhibitory effect on SGLT2, but is approximately 20 and 40 times more effective at inhibiting SGLT1 than canagliflozin and dapagliflozin respectively (253-255). In patients with type 2 diabetes treated with metformin, the addition of sotagliflozin had positive effects on HbA1c, systolic blood pressure, weight loss and postprandial blood glucose measurements. The inhibitory effects of SGLT1 were found to originate in the gut, as people with renal failure still experienced a significant decrease in postprandial glycemia (256,257). The drug is also being studied as the first oral medication for the treatment of type 1 diabetes. The inTandem trial showed that type 1 diabetes patients receiving sotagliflozin were almost twice as likely to have an HbA1c below 7.0 without an increased risk of severe hypoglycemia. However, those receiving sotagliflozin were significantly more likely to have diabetic ketoacidosis (3% vs. 0.6%) (258).

XV. Conclusion

The marked cardio-renal protection of SGLT2 inhibitors has encouraged us to elucidate their underlying mechanisms beyond hyperglycemic control. Recent studies of their general effects on glucose, lipid and protein metabolism have provided new insights into the beneficial cardio-renal effects of this class of drugs. Interestingly, SGLT2 inhibitors can induce a fasting-like metabolic paradigm involving a metabolic switch from carbohydrate to lipid utilization and ketogenesis, thereby activating nutrient deprivation pathways and helping to maintain energy homeostasis. These metabolic improvements may partly explain the cardio-renal protective effects of SGLT2 inhibitors. Further studies are needed to elucidate obscure metabolic issues and gain a comprehensive understanding of the metabolic effects of SGLT2 inhibition and their mechanisms.

iSGLT2 has a moderate beneficial effect on atherosclerosis-related major adverse cardiovascular events, which appears to be limited to patients with atherosclerotic cardiovascular disease. However, hospitalizations for heart failure and progression of renal disease were significantly reduced, irrespective of baseline atherosclerosis risk category or history of heart failure.

BIBLIOGRAPHY

1. Saeedi P, Petersohn I, Salpea P, Malanda B, Karuranga S, Unwin N, et al. Global and regional diabetes prevalence estimates for 2019 and projections for 2030 and 2045: Results from the International Diabetes Federation Diabetes Atlas, 9th edition. Diabetes Res Clin Pract. Nov 2019;157:107843.

2 American Diabetes Association. 12. Older Adults: *Standards of Medical Care in Diabetes-2019*. Diabetes Care. Jan 1, 2019;42(Supplement_1):S139-47.

3 World Health Organization. Diabetes facts sheet. 2018.

4 Zerga AA, Bezabih AM. Metabolic syndrome and lifestyle factors among type 2 diabetes mellitus patients in Dessie Referral Hospital, Amhara region, Ethiopia. Magni P, editor. PLOS ONE. Nov 2, 2020;15(11):e0241432.

5. Birkeland KI, Bodegard J, Eriksson JW, Norhammar A, Haller H, Linssen GCM, et al. Heart failure and chronic kidney disease manifestation and mortality risk associations in type 2 diabetes: A large multinational cohort study. Diabetes Obes Metab. Sept 2020;22(9):1607-18.

6. Yong J, Johnson JD, Arvan P, Han J, Kaufman RJ. Therapeutic opportunities for pancreatic β-cell ER stress in diabetes mellitus. Nat Rev Endocrinol. August 2021;17(8):455-67.

7. Kasznicki J, Drzewoski J (2014) State of the art paper heart failure in the diabetic population-pathophysiology, diagnosis and management. Arch Med Sci 3:546-556. https://doi.org/10.5114/aoms. 2014.43748.

8. Dandamudi S, Slusser J, Mahoney DW, Redfield MM, Rodeheffer RJ, Chen HH (2014) The prevalence of diabetic cardiomyopathy: a population-based study in Olmsted County, Minnesota. J Card Fail 20:304-309. https://doi.org/10.1016/j.cardfail.2014.02.007.

9. Isfort M, Stevens SCW, Schaffer S, Jong CJ, Wold LE (2014) Metabolic dysfunction in diabetic cardiomyopathy. Heart Fail Rev 19:35-48. https://doi.org/10.1007/s10741-013-9377-8.

10. Artasensi A, Pedretti A, Vistoli G, Fumagalli L. Type 2 Diabetes Mellitus: A Review of Multi-Target Drugs. Molecules. Apr 23, 2020;25(8):1987.

11. Adeghate EA, Kalász H, Al Jaberi S, Adeghate J, Tekes K. Tackling type 2 diabetes-associated cardiovascular and renal comorbidities: a key challenge for drug development. Expert Opin Investig Drugs. 1 Feb 2021;30(2):85-93.

12. Barutta F, Bernardi S, Gargiulo G, Durazzo M, Gruden G. SGLT2 inhibition to address the unmet needs in diabetic nephropathy. Diabetes Metab Res Rev [Internet]. oct 2019 [cited June 17, 2023];35(7). Available from: https://onlinelibrary.wiley.com/doi/10.1002/dmrr.3171

13. Chao EC. SGLT-2 Inhibitors: A New Mechanism for Glycemic Control. Clin Diabetes. Jan 1, 2014;32(1):4-11.

14. Matthew CR. A. Standars of medical care in diabetes ADA. Am Diabetes Assoc. 2020;42(479):960-1010.

15. Garber AJ, Handelsman Y, Grunberger G, Einhorn D, Abrahamson MJ, Barzilay JI, et al. Consensus Statement by the American Association of Clinical Endocrinologists and American College of Endocrinology on the Comprehensive Type 2 Diabetes Management Algorithm - 2020 Executive Summary. Endocr Pract. Jan 2020;26(1):107-39.

16. Zinman B, Wanner C, Lachin JM, Fitchett D, Bluhmki E, Hantel S, et al. Empagliflozin, Cardiovascular Outcomes, and Mortality in Type 2 Diabetes. N Engl J Med. Nov 26, 2015;373(22):2117-28.

17. Packer M, Anker SD, Butler J, Filippatos G, Pocock SJ, Carson P, et al. Cardiovascular and Renal Outcomes with Empagliflozin in Heart Failure. N Engl J Med. Oct 8, 2020;383(15):1413-24.

18. Vallon V, Thomson SC. The tubular hypothesis of nephron filtration and diabetic kidney disease. Nat Rev Nephrol. June 2020;16(6):317-36.

19. Bertero E, Prates Roma L, Ameri P, Maack C. Cardiac effects of SGLT2 inhibitors: the sodium hypothesis. Cardiovasc Res. 1 Jan 2018;114(1):12-8.

20 Ferrannini E, Mark M, Mayoux E. CV Protection in the EMPA-REG OUTCOME Trial: A "Thrifty Substrate" Hypothesis. Diabetes Care. 1 Jul 2016;39(7):1108-14.

21. Marton A, Kaneko T, Kovalik JP, Yasui A, Nishiyama A, Kitada K, et al. Organ protection by SGLT2 inhibitors: role of metabolic energy and water conservation. Nat Rev Nephrol. Jan 2021;17(1):65-77.

22 Hanahan D, Weinberg RA. Hallmarks of Cancer: The Next Generation. Cell. March 2011;144(5):646-74.

23. Cheng CF, Ku HC, Lin H. PGC-1α as a Pivotal Factor in Lipid and Metabolic Regulation. Int J Mol Sci. 2 Nov 2018;19(11):3447.

24. Li Y, Sha Z, Peng H. Metabolic Reprogramming in Kidney Diseases: Evidence and Therapeutic Opportunities. Anglani F, editor. Int J Nephrol. 25 Oct 2021;2021:1-6.

25. Li Z, Lu S, Li X. The role of metabolic reprogramming in tubular epithelial cells during the progression of acute kidney injury. Cell Mol Life Sci. August 2021;78(15):5731-41.

26 Gyimesi G, Pujol-Gimenez J, Kanai Y, Hediger MA. Sodium-coupled glucose transport, the SLC5 family, and therapeutically relevant inhibitors: from molecular discovery to clinical application. Pflugers Arch. 2020;472:1177-1206.

27. Cowie MR, Fisher M. SGLT2 inhibitors: mechanisms of cardiovascular benefit beyond glycaemic control. Nat Rev Cardiol. 2020;17:761-772.

28. Vallon V, Verma S. Effects of SGLT2 inhibitors on kidney and card.

29. Takeuchi T, Dohi K, Omori T, et al. Diuretic effects of sodium-glucose cotransporter 2 inhibitor in patients with type 2 diabetes mellitus and heart failure. Int J Cardiol. 2015;201:1-3. Erratum in: Int J Cardiol 2016; 206: 173.

30. Sano M. A new class of drugs for heart failure: SGLT2 inhibitors reduce sympathetic overactivity. J Cardiol. 2018;71:471-476.

31. Vallon V, Thomson SC. The tubular hypothesis of nephron filtration and diabetic kidney disease. Nat Rev Nephrol. 2020;16:317-336.

32. Packer M. Mechanisms leading to differential hypoxia-inducible factor signaling in the diabetic kidney: modulation by SGLT2 inhibitors and hypoxia mimetics. Am J Kidney Dis. 2021;77:280-286.

33. Bell RM, Yellon DM. SGLT2 inhibitors: hypotheses on the mechanism of cardiovascular protection. Lancet Diabetes Endocrinol. 2018;6:435-437.

34. Yu YW, Que JQ, Liu S, et al. Sodium-glucose co-transporter-2 inhibitor of dapagliflozin attenuates myocardial ischemia/reperfusion injury by limiting NLRP3 inflammasome activation and modulating autophagy. Front Cardiovasc Med. 2.

35. Filippatos TD, Liontos A, Papakitsou I, Elisaf MS. SGLT2 Inhibitors and Cardioprotection: A Matter of Debate and Multiple Hypotheses. Postgrad Med 2019;131:82-8.

36 Ferrannini E, Mark M, Mayoux E. CV protection in the EMPA-REG OUTCOME trial: a "thrifty substrate" hypothesis. Diabetes Care. 2016;39:1108-1114.

37 Chen HY, Huang JY, Siao WZ, Jong GP. The Association between SGLT2 Inhibitors and New-Onset Arrhythmias: A Nationwide Population-Based Longitudinal Cohort Study. Cardiovasc Diabetol 2020;19:73.

38. Yildiz M, Esenboğa K, Oktay AA. Hypertension and diabetes mellitus: highlights of a complex relationship. Curr Opin Cardiol. July 2020;35(4):397-404.

39. Lazarte J, Hegele RA. Dyslipidemia Management in Adults With Diabetes. Can J Diabetes. Feb 2020;44(1):53-60.

40. Storgaard H, Gluud LL, Bennett C, Grøndahl MF, Christensen MB, Knop FK, et al. Benefits and Harms of Sodium-Glucose Co-Transporter 2 Inhibitors in Patients with Type 2 Diabetes: A Systematic Review and Meta-Analysis. Barengo NC, editor. PLOS ONE. Nov 11, 2016;11(11):e0166125.

41. Zhang X, Zhu Q, Chen Y, Li X, Chen F, Huang J, et al. Cardiovascular Safety, Long-Term Noncardiovascular Safety, and Efficacy of Sodium-Glucose Cotransporter 2 Inhibitors in Patients With Type 2 Diabetes

Mellitus: A Systemic Review and Meta-Analysis With Trial Sequential Analysis. J Am Heart Assoc. Jan 23, 2018;7(2):e007165.

42. Borghi C, Rosei EA, Bardin T, Dawson J, Dominiczak A, Kielstein JT, et al. Serum uric acid and the risk of cardiovascular and renal disease. J Hypertens. sept 2015;33(9):1729-41.

43. Bailey CJ, Gross JL, Hennicken D, Iqbal N, Mansfield TA, List JF. Dapagliflozin add-on to metformin in type 2 diabetes inadequately controlled with metformin: a randomized, double-blind, placebo-controlled 102-week trial. BMC Med. Dec 2013;11(1):43.

44. Bailey CJ, Gross JL, Pieters A, Bastien A, List JF. Effect of dapagliflozin in patients with type 2 diabetes who have inadequate glycaemic control with metformin: a randomised, double-blind, placebo-controlled trial. The Lancet. June 2010;375(9733):2223-33.

45. McCormick N et al. Comparative effectiveness of sodium-glucose cotransporter-2 inhibitors for recurrent gout flares and gout-primary emergency department visits and hospitalizations. A general population cohort study. Ann Intern Med 2023 ; 176 : 1067-80.

46. Harrison SL, Lane DA, Banach M, Mastej M, Kasperczyk S, Jóźwiak JJ, et al. Lipid levels, atrial fibrillation and the impact of age: results from the LIPIDOGRAM2015 study. Atherosclerosis. 2020;312:16–22.

47. Ding M, Wennberg A, Gigante B, Walldius G, Hammar N, Modig K Lipid levels in midlife and risk of atrial fibrillation over 3 decades-experience from the Swedish AMORIS cohort: a cohort study. PLoS Med. 2022;19(8):e1004044.

48. Karamichalakis N, Kolovos V, Paraskevaidis I, Tsougos E. A New Hope: sodiumglucose Cotransporter-2 inhibition to prevent Atrial Fibrillation. J Cardiovasc Dev Dis. 2022;9(8).

49. Yang KC, Dudley SC Jr. Oxidative stress and atrial fibrillation: finding a missing piece to the puzzle. Circulation. 2013;128(16):1724-6.

50. Welty FK. How do elevated triglycerides and low HDL-cholesterol affect inflammation and atherothrombosis? Curr Cardiol Rep. 2013;15(9):400.

51. Lind V, Hammar N, Lundman P, Friberg L, Talbäck M, Walldius G, et al. Impaired fasting glucose: a risk factor for atrial fibrillation and Heart Failure. Cardiovasc Diabetol. 2021;20(1):227.

52. Zaccardi F, Webb DR, Htike ZZ, Youssef D, Khunti K, Davies MJ. Efficacy and safety of sodium-glucose co-transporter-2 inhibitors in type 2 diabetes mellitus: systematic review and network meta-analysis. Diabetes Obes Metab. August 2016;18(8):783-94.

53. Zelniker TA, Wiviott SD, Raz I, Im K, Goodrich EL, Bonaca MP, et al. SGLT2 inhibitors for primary and secondary prevention of cardiovascular and renal outcomes in type 2 diabetes: a systematic review and meta-analysis of cardiovascular outcome trials. The Lancet. Jan 2019;393(10166):31-9.

54. McMurray JJV, Solomon SD, Inzucchi SE, Køber L, Kosiborod MN, Martinez FA, et al. Dapagliflozin in Patients with Heart Failure and Reduced Ejection Fraction. N Engl J Med. Nov 21, 2019;381(21):1995-2008.

55. Bhatt DL, Szarek M, Steg PG, Cannon CP, Leiter LA, McGuire DK, et al. Sotagliflozin in Patients with Diabetes and Recent Worsening Heart Failure. N Engl J Med. Jan 14, 2021;384(2):117-28.

56. Bhatt DL, Szarek M, Pitt B, Cannon CP, Leiter LA, McGuire DK, et al. Sotagliflozin in Patients with Diabetes and Chronic Kidney Disease. N Engl J Med. Jan 14, 2021;384(2):129-39.

57. Kosiborod MN, Jhund PS, Docherty KF, Diez M, Petrie MC, Verma S, Nicolau JC, Merkely B , Kitakaze M, DeMets DL, Inzucchi SE, Kober L, Martinez FA, Ponikowski P, Sabatine MS, Solomon SD, Bengtsson O, Lindholm D, Niklasson A, Sjostrand M, Langkilde AM, McMurray JJV. Effects of dapaglifozin on symptoms, function, and quality of life in patients with heart failure and reduced ejection fraction: results from the DAPA-HF trial. Circulation. 2020;141:90-9.

58. Packer M, Anker SD, Butler J, Filippatos G, Pocock SJ, Carson P, Januzzi J, Verma S, Tsutsui H, Brueckmann M, Jamal W, Kimura K, Schnee J, Zeller C, Cotton D, Bocchi E, Bohm M, Choi DJ, Chopra V, Chuquiure E, Giannetti N, Janssens S, Zhang J, Gonzalez Juanatey JR, Kaul S, Brunner-La Rocca HP, Merkely B, Nicholls SJ, Perrone S, Pina I, Ponikowski P, Sattar N, Senni M, Seronde MF, Spinar J, Squire I, Taddei S, Wanner C, Zannad F, EMPEROR_Reduced Trial Investigators.

Cardiovascular and renal outcomes with empaglifozin in heart failure. N Engl J Med. 2020;383:1413-24.

59. Anker SD, Butler J, Filippatos G, Ferreira JP, Bocchi E, Böhm M, et al. Empagliflozin in Heart Failure with a Preserved Ejection Fraction. N Engl J Med. 14 Oct 2021;385(16):1451-61.

60. Williams DM, Evans M. Dapagliflozin for Heart Failure with Preserved Ejection Fraction: Will the DELIVER Study Deliver? Diabetes Ther. Oct 2020;11(10):2207-19.

61. Heerspink HJL, Stefánsson BV, Correa-Rotter R, Chertow GM, Greene T, Hou FF, et al. Dapagliflozin in Patients with Chronic Kidney Disease. N Engl J Med. 8 Oct 2020;383(15):1436-46.

62 Mazidi M, Rezaie P, Gao H, Kengne AP. Effect of Sodium-Glucose Cotransport-2 Inhibitors on Blood Pressure in People With Type 2 Diabetes Mellitus: A Systematic Review and Meta-Analysis of 43 Randomized Control Trials With 22,528 Patients. J Am Heart Assoc. Nov 6, 2017;6(6):e004007.

63. Wiviott SD, Raz I, Bonaca MP, Mosenzon O, Kato ET, Cahn A, et al. Dapagliflozin and Cardiovascular Outcomes in Type 2 Diabetes. N Engl J Med. Jan 24, 2019;380(4):347-57.

64. Almaimani M, Sridhar VS, Cherney DZI. Sodium-glucose cotransporter 2 inhibition in non-diabetic kidney disease. Curr Opin Nephrol Hypertens. Sept 2021;30(5):474-81.

65. Honka H, Solis-Herrera C, Triplitt C, Norton L, Butler J, DeFronzo RA. Therapeutic manipulation of myocardial metabolism: JACC State-of-the-Art Review. J Am Coll Cardiol. 2021;77:2022-2039.

66. Lopaschuk GD, Karwi QG, Tian R, Wende AR, Abel ED. Cardiac energy metabolism in heart failure. Circ Res. 2021;128:1487-1513.

67 Schulze PC, Wu JMF. Ketone bodies for the starving heart. Nat Metab. 2020;2:1183-1185.

68. Neinast MD, Jang C, Hui S, et al. Quantitative analysis of the whole-body metabolic fate of branched-chain amino acids. Cell Metab. 2019;29:417-429.e4.

69. Bertero E, Maack C. Metabolic remodelling in heart failure. Nat Rev Cardiol. 2018;15:457-470.

70. Davogustto GE, Salazar RL, Vasquez HG, et al. Metabolic remodeling precedes mTORC1-mediated cardiac hypertrophy. J Mol Cell Cardiol. 2021;158:115-127.

71. Bedi Jr KC, Snyder NW, Brandimarto J, et al. Evidence for intramyocardial disruption of lipid metabolism and increased myocardial ketone utilization in advanced human heart failure. Circulation. 2016;133:706-716.

72. Murashige D, Jang C, Neinast M, et al. Comprehensive quantification of fuel use by the failing and nonfailing human heart. Science. 2020;370:364-368.

73. Deng Y, Xie M, Li Q, et al. Targeting mitochondria-inflammation circuit by b-hydroxybutyrate mitigates hFpEF. Circ Res. 2021;128:232-245.

74. Neinast M, Murashige D, Arany Z. Branched chain amino acids. Annu Rev Physiol. 2019;81:139-164.

75. Wang W, Zhang F, Xia Y, et al. Defective branched chain amino acid catabolism contributes to cardiac dysfunction and remodeling following myocardial infarction. Am J Physiol Heart Circ Physiol. 2016;311:H1160-H1169.

76. Chen M, Gao C, Yu J, et al. Therapeutic effect of targeting branched-chain amino acid catabolic flux in pressure-overload induced heart failure. J Am Heart Assoc. 2019;8:e011625.

77. Uddin GM, Zhang L, Shah S, et al. Impaired branched chain amino acid oxidation contributes to cardiac insulin resistance in heart failure. Cardiovasc Diabetol. 2019;18:86.

78. D'Onofrio N, Servillo L, Balestrieri ML. SIRT1 and SIRT6 signaling pathways in cardiovascular disease protection. Antioxid Redox Signal. 2018;28:711-732.

79. Herzig S, Shaw RJ. AMPK: guardian of metabolism and mitochondria.

80. Clark AJ, Parikh SM. Targeting energy pathways in kidney disease: the roles of sirtuins, AMPK, and PGC1a. Kidney Int. 2021;99:828- 840.

81 Bhargava P, Schnellmann RG. Mitochondrial energetics in the kidney. Nat Rev Nephrol. oct 2017;13(10):629-46.

82. Cargill K, Sims-Lucas S. Metabolic requirements of the nephron. Pediatr Nephrol. Jan 2020;35(1):1-8.

83. 0 Scholz H, Felix J. Boivin, Kai M. Schmidt-Ott, Sebastian Bachmann, Kai-Uwe Eckardt, Ute I. Scholl & Pontus B. Persson. Kidney physiology and susceptibility to acute kidney injury: implications for renoprotection. Nat Rev Nephrol. 2021;(17):335-49.

84 Chen Y, Fry BC, Layton AT. Modeling glucose metabolism and lactate production in the kidney. Math Biosci. jul 2017;289:116-29.

85. Lin YC, Chang YH, Yang SY, Wu KD, Chu TS. Update of pathophysiology and management of diabetic kidney disease. J Formos Med Assoc. August 2018;117(8):662-75.

86. Sas KM, Kayampilly P, Byun J, Nair V, Hinder LM, Hur J, et al. Tissue-specific metabolic reprogramming drives nutrient flux in diabetic complications. JCI Insight [Internet]. 22 Sep 2016 [cited 9 Jul 2023];1(15). Available from: https://insight.jci.org/articles/view/86976

87. Wang XX, Levı J, Luo Y, Myakala K, Herman-Edelstein M, Qiu L, et al. SGLT2 Protein Expression Is Increased in Human Diabetic Nephropathy. J Biol Chem. March 2017;292(13):5335-48.

88. Kogot-Levin A, Hinden L, Riahi Y, Israeli T, Tirosh B, Cerasi E, et al. Proximal Tubule mTORC1 Is a Central Player in the Pathophysiology of Diabetic Nephropathy and Its Correction by SGLT2 Inhibitors. Cell Rep. July 2020;32(4):107954.

89. Kidokoro K, Cherney DZI, Bozovic A, Nagasu H, Satoh M, Kanda E, et al. Evaluation of Glomerular Hemodynamic Function by Empagliflozin in Diabetic Mice Using In Vivo Imaging. Circulation. 23 Jul 2019;140(4):303-15.

90. Van Bommel EJM, Muskiet MHA, Van Baar MJB, Tonneijck L, Smits MM, Emanuel AL, et al. The renal hemodynamic effects of the SGLT2 inhibitor dapagliflozin are caused by post-glomerular vasodilation

rather than pre-glomerular vasoconstriction in metformin-treated patients with type 2 diabetes in the randomized, double-blind RED trial. Kidney Int. Jan 2020;97(1):202-12.

91. Heerspink HJL, Kosiborod M, Inzucchi SE, Cherney DZI. Renoprotective effects of sodium-glucose cotransporter-2 inhibitors. Kidney Int. Jul 2018;94(1):26-39.

92. Gilbert RE. Proximal Tubulopathy: Prime Mover and Key Therapeutic Target in Diabetic Kidney Disease. Diabetes. Apr 1, 2017;66(4):791-800.

93. Kim J, Plitman E, Nakajima S, Alshehri Y, Iwata Y, Chung JK, et al. Modulation of brain activity with transcranial direct current stimulation: Targeting regions implicated in impaired illness awareness in schizophrenia. Eur Psychiatry. sept 2019;61:63-71.

94. Cai T, Ke Q, Fang Y, Wen P, Chen H, Yuan Q, et al. Sodium-glucose cotransporter 2 inhibition suppresses HIF-1α-mediated metabolic switch from lipid oxidation to glycolysis in kidney tubule cells of diabetic mice. Cell Death Dis. May 22, 2020;11(5):390.

95. Lieben L. Lipid toxicity drives renal disease. Nat Rev Nephrol. Apr 2017;13(4):194-194.

96. Li ZL, Lv LL, Tang TT, Wang B, Feng Y, Zhou LT, et al. HIF-1α inducing exosomal microRNA-23a expression mediates the cross-talk between tubular epithelial cells and macrophages in tubulointerstitial inflammation. Kidney Int. Feb 2019;95(2):388-404.

97. Kim Y, Park CW. Adenosine monophosphate-activated protein kinase in diabetic nephropathy. Kidney Res Clin Pract. June 2016;35(2):69-77.

98. Fantus D, Rogers NM, Grahammer F, Huber TB, Thomson AW. Roles of mTOR complexes in the kidney: implications for renal disease and transplantation. Nat Rev Nephrol. oct 2016;12(10):587-609.

99. Yasuda-Yamahara M, Kume S, Maegawa H. Roles of mTOR in Diabetic Kidney Disease. Antioxidants. 22 Feb 2021;10(2):321.

100. Ferrannini G, Hach T, Crowe S, Sanghvi A, Hall KD, Ferrannini E. Energy balance after sodium-glucose cotransporter 2 inhibition. Diabetes Care. 2015;38:1730-1735.

101. Al Jobori H, Daniele G, Adams J, et al. Empagliflozin treatment is associated with improved b-cell function in type 2 diabetes mellitus. J Clin Endocrinol Metab. 2018;103:1402-1407.

102 Kalra S, Gupta Y. The insulin:glucagon ratio and the choice of glucose-lowering drugs. Diabetes Ther. 2016;7:1-9.

103 Wolf P, Fellinger P, Pfleger L, et al. Gluconeogenesis, but not glycogenolysis, contributes to the increase in endogenous glucose production by SGLT-2 inhibition. D.

104 Matsuba R, Matsuba I, Shimokawa M, Nagai Y, Tanaka Y. Tofogliflozin decreases body fat mass and improves peripheral insulin resistance. Diabetes Obes Metab. 2018;20:1311-1315.

105. Tanaka S, Sugiura Y, Saito H, et al. Sodium-glucose cotransporter 2 inhibition normalizes glucose metabolism and suppresses oxida_tive stress in the kidneys of diabetic mice. Kidney Int. 2018;94:912- 925.

106. Ferrannini E, Baldi S, Frascerra S, et al. Shift to fatty substrate utilization in response to sodium-glucose cotransporter 2 inhibition in subjects without diabetes and patients with type 2 diabetes. Diabetes. 2016;65:1190-1195.

107. Verma S, Rawat S, Ho KL, et al. Empagliflozin increases cardiac energy production in diabetes: novel translational insights into the heart failure benefits of SGLT2 inhibitors. JACC Basic Transl Sci. 2018;3:575-587.

108. Koyani CN, Plastira I, Sourij H, et al. Empagliflozin protects heart from inflammation and energy depletion via AMPK activation. Pharmacol Res. 2020;158:104870.

109. Xu L, Nagata N, Nagashimada M, et al. SGLT2 Inhibition by empagliflozin promotes fat utilization and browning and attenuates inflammation and insulin resistance by polarizing M2 macrophages in diet-induced obese mice. EBioMedicine. 2017;20:137-149.

110. Swe MT, Thongnak L, Jaikumkao K, Pongchaidecha A, Chatsudthipong V, Lungkaphin A. Dapagliflozin not only improves hepatic injury and pancreatic endoplasmic reticulum stress, but also induces hepatic gluconeogenic enzymes expression in obese rats. Clin Sci (Lond). 2019;133:2415-2430.

111. Mancini SJ, Boyd D, Katwan OJ, et al. Canagliflozin inhibits interleukin-1b-stimulated cytokine and chemokine secretion in vascular endothelial cells by AMP-activated protein kinase-dependent and -independent mechanisms. Sci Rep. 2018;8:5276.

112. Bessho R, Takiyama Y, Takiyama T, et al. Hypoxia-inducible factor1a is the therapeutic target of the SGLT2 inhibitor for diabetic nephropathy. Sci Rep. 2019;9:14754.

113 Fantus D, Rogers NM, Grahammer F, Huber TB, Thomson AW. Roles of mTOR complexes in the kidney: implications for renal disease and transplantation. Nat Rev Nephrol. 2016;12:587-609.

114. Blackwood EA, Hofmann C, Santo Domingo M, et al. ATF6 regulates cardiac hypertrophy by transcriptional induction of the mTORC1 activator, Rheb. Circ Res. 2019;124:79-93.

115. Kogot-Levin A, Hinden L, Riahi Y, et al. Proximal tubule mTORC1 is a central player in the pathophysiology of diabetic nephropathy and its correction by SGLT2 Inhibitors. Cell Rep. 2020;32:107954.

116. Sun X, Han F, Lu Q, et al. Empagliflozin ameliorates obesityrelated cardiac dysfunction by regulating sestrin2-mediated AMPK-mTOR Signaling and redox homeostasis in high-fat dietinduced obese mice. Diabetes. 2020;69:1292-1305.

117. Ren C, Sun K, Zhang Y, et al. Sodium-glucose cotransporter-2 inhibitor empagliflozin ameliorates sunitinib-induced cardiac dysfunction via regulation of AMPK-mTOR signaling pathway-mediated autophagy. Front Pharmacol. 2021;12:664181.

118. Xu J, Kitada M, Ogura Y, Liu H, Koya D. Dapagliflozin restores impaired autophagy and suppresses inflammation in high glucosetreated HK-2 cells. Cells. 2021;10:145.

119. Tomita I, Kume S, Sugahara S, et al. SGLT2 inhibition mediates protection from diabetic kidney disease by promoting ketone bodyinduced mTORC1 inhibition. Cell Metab. 2020;32:404-419. .e6.

120. Wiviott SD, Raz I, Bonaca MP, Mosenzon O, Kato ET, Cahn A, et al. Dapagliflozin and Cardiovascular Outcomes in Type 2 Diabetes. N Engl J Med. Jan 24, 2019;380(4):347-57.

121. Neal B, Perkovic V, Mahaffey KW, De Zeeuw D, Fulcher G, Erondu N, et al. Canagliflozin and Cardiovascular and Renal Events in Type 2 Diabetes. N Engl J Med. August 17, 2017;377(7):644-57.

122. Perkovic V, Jardine MJ, Neal B, Bompoint S, Heerspink HJL, Charytan DM, et al. Canagliflozin and Renal Outcomes in Type 2 Diabetes and Nephropathy. N Engl J Med. June 13, 2019;380(24):2295-306.

123. Rajasekeran H, Cherney DZ, Lovshin JA. Do effects of sodium-glucose cotransporter-2 inhibitors in patients with diabetes give insight into potential use in non-diabetic kidney disease: Curr Opin Nephrol Hypertens. sept 2017;26(5):358-67.

124 Dekkers CCJ, Gansevoort RT, Heerspink HJL. New Diabetes Therapies and Diabetic Kidney Disease Progression: the Role of SGLT-2 Inhibitors. Curr Diab Rep. May 2018;18(5):27.

125. Heerspink HJL, Stefansson BV, Chertow GM, Correa-Rotter R, Greene T, Hou FF, et al. Rationale and protocol of the Dapagliflozin And Prevention of Adverse outcomes in Chronic Kidney Disease (DAPA-CKD) randomized controlled trial. Nephrol Dial Transplant. Feb 1, 2020;35(2):274-82.

126. Heerspink HJL, Perkins BA, Fitchett DH, Husain M, Cherney DZI. Sodium Glucose Cotransporter 2 Inhibitors in the Treatment of Diabetes Mellitus: Cardiovascular and Kidney Effects, Potential Mechanisms, and Clinical Applications. Circulation. Sep 6, 2016;134(10):752-72.

127. Lundkvist P, Sjöström CD, Amini S, Pereira MJ, Johnsson E, Eriksson JW. Dapagliflozin once-daily and exenatide once-weekly dual therapy: A 24-week randomized, placebo-controlled, phase II study examining effects on body weight and prediabetes in obese adults without diabetes: Lundkvist et al. Diabetes Obes Metab. jan 2017;19(1):49-60.

128. Komoroski B, Vachharajani N, Boulton D, Kornhauser D, Geraldes M, Li L, et al. Dapagliflozin, a Novel SGLT2 Inhibitor, Induces Dose-Dependent Glucosuria in Healthy Subjects. Clin Pharmacol Ther. May 2009;85(5):520-6.

129. Al Jobori H, Daniele G, Adams J, Cersosimo E, Triplitt C, DeFronzo RA, et al. Determinants of the increase in ketone concentration during

SGLT2 inhibition in NGT, IFG and T2DM patients. Diabetes Obes Metab. June 2017;19(6):809-13.

130. Dekkers CCJ, Wheeler DC, Sjöström CD, Stefansson BV, Cain V, Heerspink HJL. Effects of the sodium-glucose co-transporter 2 inhibitor dapagliflozin in patients with type 2 diabetes and Stages 3b-4 chronic kidney disease. Nephrol Dial Transplant. 1 Nov 2018;33(11):2005-11.

131. Pleros C, Stamataki E, Papadaki A, Damianakis N, Poulidaki R, Gakiopoulou C, et al. Dapagliflozin as a cause of acute tubular necrosis with heavy consequences: a case report. CEN Case Rep. May 2018;7(1):17-20.

132. Perkovic V, De Zeeuw D, Mahaffey KW, Fulcher G, Erondu N, Shaw W, et al. Canagliflozin and renal outcomes in type 2 diabetes: results from the CANVAS Program randomised clinical trials. Lancet Diabetes Endocrinol. Sept 2018;6(9):691-704.

133. McMurray J. Dapagliflozin in patients with heart failure and reduced ejection fraction (DAPA-HF). Presented at the European Society for Cardiology Congress 2019, Paris, France. Sep 1, 2019;

134. Heerspink HJL, Desai M, Jardine M, Balis D, Meininger G, Perkovic V. Canagliflozin Slows Progression of Renal Function Decline Independently of Glycemic Effects. J Am Soc Nephrol. jan 2017;28(1):368-75.

135. Holtkamp FA, De Zeeuw D, Thomas MC, Cooper ME, De Graeff PA, Hillege HJL, et al. An acute fall in estimated glomerular filtration rate during treatment with losartan predicts a slower decrease in long-term renal function. Kidney Int. August 2011;80(3):282-7.

136. Jardine MJ, Zhou Z, Mahaffey KW, Oshima M, Agarwal R, Bakris G, et al. Renal, Cardiovascular, and Safety Outcomes of Canagliflozin by Baseline Kidney Function: A Secondary Analysis of the CREDENCE Randomized Trial. J Am Soc Nephrol. May 2020;31(5):1128-39.

137. Brenner BM, Ballermann BJ, Gunning ME, Zeidel ML. Diverse biological actions of atrial natriuretic peptide. Physiol Rev. 1 Jul 1990;70(3):665-99.

138. Cherney DZI, Perkins BA, Soleymanlou N, Maione M, Lai V, Lee A, et al. Renal Hemodynamic Effect of Sodium-Glucose Cotransporter 2

Inhibition in Patients With Type 1 Diabetes Mellitus. Circulation. Feb 4, 2014;129(5):587-97.

139. Ortola FV, Ballermann BJ, Anderson S, Mendez RE, Brenner BM. Elevated plasma atrial natriuretic peptide levels in diabetic rats. Potential mediator of hyperfiltration. J Clin Invest. 1 Sep 1987;80(3):670-4.

140. Chakraborty S, Galla S, Cheng X, Yeo JY, Mell B, Singh V, et al. Salt-Responsive Metabolite, β-Hydroxybutyrate, Attenuates Hypertension. Cell Rep. Oct 2018;25(3):677-689.e4.

141. Sternlicht H, Bakris GL. Blood Pressure Lowering and Sodium-Glucose Co-transporter 2 Inhibitors (SGLT2is): More Than Osmotic Diuresis. Curr Hypertens Rep. Feb 2019;21(2):12.

142. Esterline RL, Vaag A, Oscarsson J, Vora J. MECHANISMS IN ENDOCRINOLOGY: SGLT2 inhibitors: clinical benefits by restoration of normal diurnal metabolism? Eur J Endocrinol. Apr 2018;178(4):R113-25.

143. Fountoulaki, K.; Ventoulis, I.; Drokou, A.; Georgarakou, K.; Parissis, J.; Polyzogopoulou, E. Emergency Department Risk Assessment and Disposition of Acute Heart Failure Patients: Existing Evidence and Ongoing Challenges. Heart Fail. Rev. 2022; online ahead of print.

144. Arrigo, M.; Jessup, M.; Mullens, W.; Reza, N.; Shah, A.M.; Sliwa, K.; Mebazaa, A. Acute Heart Failure. Nat. Rev. Dis. Prim. 2020, 6, 16.

145. Shiraishi, Y.; Kohsaka, S.; Sato, N.; Takano, T.; Kitai, T.; Yoshikawa, T.; Matsue, Y. 9-year Trend in the Management of Acute Heart Failure in Japan: A Report from the National Consortium of Acute Heart Failure Registries. J. Am. Heart Assoc. 2018, 7, e008687.

146. Bytyçi, I.; Bajraktari, G. Mortality in Heart Failure Patients. Anatol. J. Cardiol. 2015, 15, 63.

147. Cox, Z.L.; Collins, S.P.; Aaron, M.; Hernandez, G.A.; McRae, A.T., III; Davidson, B.T.; Fowler, M.; Lindsell, C.J.; Harrell, F.E., Jr.; Jenkins, C.A. Efficacy and Safety of Dapagliflozin in Acute Heart Failure: Rationale and Design of the DICTATE-AHF Trial. Am. Heart J. 2021, 232, 116-124.

148. Buddeke, J.; Valstar, G.B.; Van Dis, I.; Visseren, F.L.J.; Rutten, F.H.; Den Ruijter, H.M.; Vaartjes, I.; Bots, M.L. Mortality after Hospital

Admission for Heart Failure: Improvement over Time, Equally Strong in Women as in Men. BMC Public Health 2020, 20, 36.

149. Tsutsui, H. Recent Advances in the Pharmacological Therapy of Chronic Heart Failure: Evidence and Guidelines. Pharmacol. Ther. 2022, 238, 108185.

150. Mullens, W.; Damman, K.; Harjola, V.; Mebazaa, A.; Brunner-La Rocca, H.; Martens, P.; Testani, J.M.; Tang, W.H.W.; Orso, F.; Rossignol, P. The Use of Diuretics in Heart Failure with Congestion-A Position Statement from the Heart Failure Association of the European Society of Cardiology. Eur. J. Heart Fail. 2019, 21, 137-155.

151. Mazza, A.; Townsend, D.M.; Torin, G.; Schiavon, L.; Camerotto, A.; Rigatelli, G.; Cuppini, S.; Minuz, P.; Rubello, D. The Role of Sacubitril/Valsartan in the Treatment of Chronic Heart Failure with Reduced Ejection Fraction in Hypertensive Patients with Comorbidities: From Clinical Trials to Real-World Settings. Biomed. Pharmacother. 2020, 130, 110596.

152. Felker, G.M.; O'Connor, C.M.; Braunwald, E. Loop Diuretics in Acute Decompensated Heart Failure: Necessary? Evil? A Necessary Evil? Circ. Heart Fail. 2009, 2, 56-62.

153. Kosiborod, M.N.; Angermann, C.E.; Collins, S.P.; Teerlink, J.R.; Ponikowski, P.; Biegus, J.; Comin-Colet, J.; Ferreira, J.P.; Mentz, R.J.; Nassif, M.E. Effects of Empagliflozin on Symptoms, Physical Limitations and Quality of Life in Patients Hospitalized for Acute Heart Failure-Results from the EMPULSE Trial. Circulation 2022, 146, 279-288.

154. Savarese, G.; Sattar, N.; Januzzi, J.; Verma, S.; Lund, L.H.; Fitchett, D.; Zeller, C.; George, J.T.; Brueckmann, M.; Ofstad, A.P. Empagliflozin Is Associated with a Lower Risk of Post-Acute Heart Failure Rehospitalization and Mortality: Insights from the EMPA-REG OUTCOME Trial. Circulation 2019, 139, 1458-1460.

155. Damman, K.; Beusekamp, J.C.; Boorsma, E.M.; Swart, H.P.; Smilde, T.D.J.; Elvan, A.; van Eck, J.W.M.; Heerspink, H.J.L.; Voors, A.A. Randomized, Double-blind, Placebo-controlled, Multicentre Pilot Study on the Effects of Empagliflozin on Clinical Outcomes in Patients with Acute Decompensated Heart Failure (EMPA-RESPONSE-AHF). Eur. J. Heart Fail. 2020, 22, 713-722.

156. Voors, A.A.; Angermann, C.E.; Teerlink, J.R.; Collins, S.P.; Kosiborod, M.; Biegus, J.; Ferreira, J.P.; Nassif, M.E.; Psotka, M.A.; Tromp, J. The SGLT2 Inhibitor Empagliflozin in Patients Hospitalized for Acute Heart Failure: A Multinational Randomized Trial. Nat. Med. 2022, 28, 568-574.

157. Tromp, J.; Ponikowski, P.; Salsali, A.; Angermann, C.E.; Biegus, J.; Blatchford, J.; Collins, S.P.; Ferreira, J.P.; Grauer, C.; Kosiborod, M. Sodium-Glucose Co-transporter 2 Inhibition in Patients Hospitalized for Acute Decompensated Heart Failure: Rationale for and Design of the EMPULSE Trial. Eur. J. Heart Fail. 2021, 23, 826-834.

158. Spertus, J.A.; Birmingham, M.C.; Nassif, M.; Damaraju, C.V.; Abbate, A.; Butler, J.; Lanfear, D.E.; Lingvay, I.; Kosiborod, M.N.; Januzzi, J.L. The SGLT2 Inhibitor Canagliflozin in Heart Failure: The CHIEF-HF Remote, Patient-Centered Randomized Trial. Nat. Med. 2022, 28, 809-813.

159. Tamaki, S.; Yamada, T.; Watanabe, T.; Morita, T.; Furukawa, Y.; Kawasaki, M.; Kikuchi, A.; Kawai, T.; Seo, M.; Abe, M. Effect of Empagliflozin as an Add-on Therapy on Decongestion and Renal Function in Patients with Diabetes Hospitalized for Acute Decompensated Heart Failure: A Prospective Randomized Controlled Study. Circ. Heart Fail. 2021, 14, e007048.

160. Chewcharat A, Prasitlumkum N, Thongprayoon C, Bathini T, Medaura J, Vallabhajosyula S, et al. Efficacy and Safety of SGLT-2 Inhibitors for Treatment of Diabetes Mellitus among Kidney Transplant Patients: A Systematic Review and Meta-Analysis. Med Sci Basel Switz. 17 Nov 2020;8(4):47.

161. Heerspink HJL. Sodium glucose co-transporter 2 inhibition: a new avenue to protect the kidney. Nephrol Dial Transplant. Dec 1, 2019;34(12):2015-7.

162 Vergara A, Jacobs-Cachá C, Soler MJ. Sodium-glucose cotransporter inhibitors: beyond glycaemic control. Clin Kidney J. June 1, 2019;12(3):322-5.

163. Clar C, Gill JA, Court R, Waugh N. Systematic review of SGLT2 receptor inhibitors in dual or triple therapy in type 2 diabetes. BMJ Open. 2012;2(5):e001007.

164. Musso G, Gambino R, Cassader M, Pagano G. A novel approach to control hyperglycemia in type 2 diabetes: Sodium glucose co-transport (SGLT) inhibitors. Systematic review and meta-analysis of randomized trials. Ann Med. June 2012;44(4):375-93.

165. Toyama T, Neuen BL, Jun M, Ohkuma T, Neal B, Jardine MJ, et al. Effect of SGLT2 inhibitors on cardiovascular, renal and safety outcomes in patients with type 2 diabetes mellitus and chronic kidney disease: A systematic review and meta-analysis. Diabetes Obes Metab. May 2019;21(5):1237-50.

166. Foote C, Perkovic V, Neal B. Effects of SGLT2 inhibitors on cardiovascular outcomes. Diab Vasc Dis Res. Apr 2012;9(2):117-23.

167. Ceriello A, Ofstad AP, Zwiener I, Kaspers S, George J, Nicolucci A. Empagliflozin reduced long-term HbA1c variability and cardiovascular death: insights from the EMPA-REG OUTCOME trial. Cardiovasc Diabetol. Dec 2020;19(1):176.

168. Yaribeygi H, Atkin SL, Sahebkar A. Mechanistic effects of SGLT2 inhibition on blood pressure in diabetes. Diabetes Metab Syndr Clin Res Rev. March 2019;13(2):1679-83.

169. Weir MR, Burgess ED, Cooper JE, Fenves AZ, Goldsmith D, McKay D, et al. Assessment and Management of Hypertension in Transplant Patients. J Am Soc Nephrol. June 2015;26(6):1248-60.

170. Halden TAS, Kvitne KE, Midtvedt K, Rajakumar L, Robertsen I, Brox J, et al. Efficacy and Safety of Empagliflozin in Renal Transplant Recipients With Posttransplant Diabetes Mellitus. Diabetes Care. June 1, 2019;42(6):1067-74.

171. Heerspink HJL, Perco P, Mulder S, Leierer J, Hansen MK, Heinzel A, et al. Canagliflozin reduces inflammation and fibrosis biomarkers: a potential mechanism of action for beneficial effects of SGLT2 inhibitors in diabetic kidney disease. Diabetologia. Jul 2019;62(7):1154-66.

172. Yaribeygi H, Simental-Mendía LE, Banach M, Bo S, Sahebkar A. The major molecular mechanisms mediating the renoprotective effects of SGLT2 inhibitors: An update. Biomed Pharmacother. Dec 2019;120:109526.

173. Hattori S. Anti-inflammatory effects of empagliflozin in patients with type 2 diabetes and insulin resistance. Diabetol Metab Syndr. Dec 2018;10(1):93.

174. Packer M. SGLT2 Inhibitors Produce Cardiorenal Benefits by Promoting Adaptive Cellular Reprogramming to Induce a State of Fasting Mimicry: A Paradigm Shift in Understanding Their Mechanism of Action. Diabetes Care. March 1, 2020;43(3):508-11.

175. Iannantuoni F, M. De Marañon A, Diaz-Morales N, Falcon R, Bañuls C, Abad-Jimenez Z, et al. The SGLT2 Inhibitor Empagliflozin Ameliorates the Inflammatory Profile in Type 2 Diabetic Patients and Promotes an Antioxidant Response in Leukocytes. J Clin Med. Nov 1, 2019;8(11):1814.

176. Wu X, Dong Y, Liu Y, Li Y, Sun Y, Wang J, et al. The prevalence and predictive factors of urinary tract infection in patients undergoing renal transplantation: A meta-analysis. Am J Infect Control. nov 2016;44(11):1261-8.

177. Liu J, Li L, Li S, Jia P, Deng K, Chen W, et al. Effects of SGLT2 inhibitors on UTIs and genital infections in type 2 diabetes mellitus: a systematic review and meta-analysis. Sci Rep. June 6, 2017;7(1):2824.

178 Peters AL, Buschur EO, Buse JB, Cohan P, Diner JC, Hirsch IB. Euglycemic Diabetic Ketoacidosis: A Potential Complication of Treatment With Sodium-Glucose Cotransporter 2 Inhibition. Diabetes Care. Sep 1, 2015;38(9):1687-93.

179 Lee PC, Ganguly S, Goh SY. Weight loss associated with sodium-glucose cotransporter-2 inhibition: a review of evidence and underlying mechanisms: SGLT2 inhibitor mediated weight loss. Obes Rev. Dec 2018;19(12):1630-41.

180. Nespoux J, Vallon V. SGLT2 inhibition and kidney protection. Clin Sci. June 29, 2018;132(12):1329-39.

181. Phadke G, Kaushal A, Tolan DR, Hahn K, Jensen T, Bjornstad P, et al. Osmotic Nephrosis and Acute Kidney Injury Associated With SGLT2 Inhibitor Use: A Case Report. Am J Kidney Dis. July 2020;76(1):144-7.

182. Opingari E, Partridge ACR, Verma S, et al. SGLT2 Inhibitors: Practical Considerations and Recommendations for Cardiologists. Curr Opin Cardiol 2018;33:676-82.

183. Scheen AJ. An update on the safety of SGLT2 inhibitors. Expert Opin Drug Saf . 2019. doi:10.1080/14740338.2019.1602116.

184. Johnsson KM , Ptaszynska A , Schmitz B , et al. Vulvovaginitis and balanitis in patients with diabetes treated with dapagliflozin. J Diabetes Complications . 2013;27(5):479–484. doi:10.1016/j.jdiacomp.2013.04.012 23806570.

185. Bailey CJ , Gross JL , Pieters A , et al. Effect of dapagliflozin in patients with type 2 diabetes who have inadequate glycaemic control with metformin: a randomised, double-blind, placebo-controlled trial. Lancet . 2010;375(9733):2223-2233. doi:10.1016/s0140-6736(10)60407-2 20609968.

186. Bode B , Stenlöf K , Harris S , et al. Long-term efficacy and safety of canagliflozin over 104 weeks in patients aged 55-80 years with type 2 diabetes. Diabetes Obesity Metab . 2015;17(3):294–303. doi:10.1111/dom.12428.

187 Scheen AJ. SGLT2 inhibitors: benefit/risk balance. Curr Diabetes Rep 2016;16:92.

188. Horii T, Oikawa Y, Kunisada N, Shimada A, Atsuda K. Real-world risk of hypoglycemia-related hospitalization in Japanese patients with type 2 diabetes using SGLT2 inhibitors: a nationwide cohort study. BMJ Open Diabetes Res Care. 2020 Nov;8(2).

189. Daniele G , Xiong J , Solis-Herrera C , et al. Dapagliflozin enhances fat oxidation and ketone production in patients with type 2 diabetes. Diabetes Care . 2016;39(11):2036-2041. doi:10.2337/dc15-2688 27561923.

190. Perry RJ , Rabin-Court A , Song JD , et al. Dehydration and insulinopenia are necessary and sufficient for euglycemic ketoacidosis in SGLT2 inhibitor-treated rats. Nat Commun . 2019;10:(1):548. doi:10.1038/s41467-019-08466-w 30602773.

191. Peters AL , Buschur EO , Buse JB , et al. Euglycemic diabetic ketoacidosis: a potential complication of treatment with sodium-

glucose cotransporter 2 inhibition. Diabetes Care . 2015;38(9):1687-1693. doi:10.2337/dc15-0843 26078479.

192. Fralick M , Schneeweiss S , Patorno E . Risk of diabetic ketoacidosis after initiation of an SGLT2 inhibitor. N Engl J Med . 2017;376(23):2300-2302. doi:10.1056/nejmc1701990 28591538.

193. Donnan JR , Grandy CA , Chibrikov E , et al. Comparative safety of the sodium glucose co-transporter 2 (SGLT2) inhibitors: a systematic review and meta-analysis. BMJ Open . 2019;9:1. doi:10.1136/bmjopen-2018-022577.

194. Saad M , Mahmoud AN , Elgendy IY , et al. Cardiovascular outcomes with sodium-glucose cotransporter-2 inhibitors in patients with type II diabetes mellitus: a meta-analysis of placebo-controlled randomized trials. Int J Cardiol . 2017;228:352-358. doi:10.1016/j.ijcard.2016.11.181 27866027.

195. Rosenstock J, Ferrannini E. Euglycemic diabetic ketoacidosis: a predictable, detectable, and preventable safety concern with SGLT2 inhibitors. Diabetes Care 2015;38:1638-42.

196. Neal B, Perkovic V, Mahaffey KW, et al. Canagliflozin and Cardiovascular and Renal Events in Type 2 Diabetes. N Engl J Med 2017;377:644-57.

197 Fadini GP, Avogaro A. SGLT2 inhibitors and amputations in the US FDA Adverse Event Reporting System. Lancet Diabetes Endocrinol. sept 2017;5(9):680-1.

198. Kaneko M , Narukawa M . Effects of sodium-glucose cotransporter 2 inhibitors on amputation, bone fracture, and cardiovascular outcomes in patients with type 2 diabetes mellitus using an alternative measure to the hazard ratio. Clin Drug Investig . 2018;39(2):179-186. doi:10.1007/s40261-018-0731-4.

199. Kohler S , Zeller C , Iliev H , et al. Safety and tolerability of empagliflozin in patients with type 2 diabetes: pooled analysis of phase I-III clinical trials. Adv Ther . 2017;34(7):1707–1726. doi:10.1007/s12325-017-0573-0 28631216.

200. Chang H-Y , Singh S , Mansour O , et al. Association between sodium-glucose cotransporter 2 inhibitors and lower extremity

amputation among patients with type 2 diabetes. JAMA Intern Med . 2018;178(9):1190-1198. doi:10.1001/jamainternmed.2018.3034 30105373.

201. Vestergaard P. Discrepancies in bone mineral density and fracture risk in patients with type 1 and type 2 diabetes-a meta-analysis. Osteoporosis Int . 2006;18(4):427–444. doi:10.1007/s00198-006-0253-4.

202. Janghorbani M , Dam RMV , Willett WC , et al. Systematic review of type 1 and type 2 diabetes mellitus and risk of fracture. Am J Epidemiol . 2007;166(5):495-505. doi:10.1093/aje/kwm106 17575306.

203. Ma L , Oei L , Jiang L , et al. Association between bone mineral density and type 2 diabetes mellitus: a meta-analysis of observational studies. Eur J Epidemiol . 2012;27(5):319-332. doi:10.1007/s10654-012-9674-x 22451239.

204. Thrailkill KM , Nyman JS , Bunn RC , et al. The impact of SGLT2 inhibitors, compared with insulin, on diabetic bone disease in a mouse model of type 1 diabetes. Bone . 2017;94:141-151. doi:10.1016/j.bone.2016.10.026 27989651.

205. Thrailkill KM , Bunn RC , Nyman JS , et al. SGLT2 inhibitor therapy improves blood glucose but does not prevent diabetic bone disease in diabetic DBA/2J male mice. Bone . 2016;82:101-107. doi:10.1016/j.bone.2015.07.025 26211996.

206. Bilezikian JP , Watts NB , Usiskin K , et al. Evaluation of bone mineral density and bone biomarkers in patients with type 2 diabetes treated with canagliflozin. J Clin Endocrinol Metab . 2016;101(1):44-51. doi:10.1210/jc.2015-1860 26580234.

207. Kohan DE , Fioretto P , Tang W , et al. Long-term study of patients with type 2 diabetes and moderate renal impairment shows that dapagliflozin reduces weight and blood pressure but does not improve glycemic control. Kidney Int . 2014;85(4):962-971. doi:10.1038/ki.2013.356 24067431.

208. Watts NB , Bilezikian JP , Usiskin K , et al. Effects of canagliflozin on fracture risk in patients with type 2 diabetes mellitus. J Clin Endocrinol Metab . 2016;101(1):157-166. doi:10.1210/jc.2015-3167 26580237.

209. Ruanpeng D , Ungprasert P , Sangtian J , et al. Sodium-glucose cotransporter 2 (SGLT2) inhibitors and fracture risk in patients with type 2 diabetes mellitus: a meta-analysis. Diabetes Metab Res Rev . 2017;33:6. doi:10.1002/dmrr.2903.

210. Ritesh J , U.S. Food and Drug Administration. Center for Drug Evaluation and Research. Dapagliflozin Clinical Pharmacology Review (Report No. 202293). Silver Spring, MD: Division of Drug Information.

211. Tikkanen I , Narko K , Zeller C , et al. Empagliflozin reduces blood pressure in patients with type 2 diabetes and hypertension. Diabetes Care . 2015;38(3):420-428. doi:10.2337/dc14-1096 25271206.

212. Wiviott SD , Raz I , Bonaca MP , et al. Dapagliflozin and cardiovascular outcomes in type 2 diabetes. N Engl J Med . 2019;380(4):347-357. doi:10.1056/nejmoa1812389 30415602.

213. Tang H , Dai Q , Shi W , Zhai S , Song Y , Han J . SGLT2 inhibitors and risk of cancer in type 2 diabetes: a systematic review and meta-analysis of randomised controlled trials. Diabetologia . 2017;60(10):1862–1872. doi:10.1007/s00125-017-4370-8 28725912.

214. Shaikh A . SGLT2 inhibitors and cancer: why further evidence is required. Diabetologia . 2017;60(12):2536–2537. doi:10.1007/s00125-017-4434-9 28905192.

215. Dicembrini I , Nreu B , Mannucci E , et al. Sodium-glucose co-transporter-2 (SGLT-2) inhibitors and cancer: a meta-analysis of randomized controlled trials. Diabetes Obesity Metab . 2019. doi:10.1111/dom.13745.

216. Häring H-U , Merker L , Seewaldt-Becker E , et al. Empagliflozin as add-on to metformin in patients with type 2 diabetes: a 24-week, randomized, double-blind, placebo-controlled trial. Diabetes Care . 2014;37(6):1650-1659. doi:10.2337/dc13-2105 24722494.

217. Roden M , Weng J , Eilbracht J , et al. Empagliflozin monotherapy with sitagliptin as an active comparator in patients with type 2 diabetes: a randomised, double-blind, placebo-controlled, phase 3 trial. Lancet Diabetes Endocrinol . 2013;1(3):208-219. doi:10.1016/s2213-8587(13)70084-6 24622369.

218. Zinman B , Wanner C , Lachin JM , et al. Empagliflozin, cardiovascular outcomes, and mortality in type 2 diabetes. N Engl J Med . 2015;373(22):2117-2128. doi:10.1056/nejmoa1504720 26378978.

219. Kovacs CS , Seshiah V , Swallow R , et al. Empagliflozin improves glycaemic and weight control as add-on therapy to pioglitazone or pioglitazone plus metformin in patients with type 2 diabetes: a 24-week, randomized, placebo-controlled trial. Diabetes Obesity Metab . 2013;16(2):147–158. doi:10.1111/dom.12188.

220. Storgaard H , Gluud LL , Bennett C , et al. Benefits and harms of sodium-glucose co-transporter 2 inhibitors in patients with type 2 diabetes: a systematic review and meta-analysis. PLoS One . 2016;11:11. doi:10.1371/journal.pone.0166125.

221. Hayashi T , Fukui T , Nakanishi N , et al. Dapagliflozin decreases small dense low-density lipoprotein-cholesterol and increases high-density lipoprotein 2-cholesterol in patients with type 2 diabetes: comparison with sitagliptin. Cardiovasc Diabetol . 2017;16:1. doi:10.1186/s12933-016-0491-5 28057001.

222. Pieber TR , Famulla S , Eilbracht J , et al. Empagliflozin as adjunct to insulin in patients with type 1 diabetes: a 4-week, randomized, placebo-controlled trial (EASE-1). Diabetes Obesity Metab . 2015;17(10):928–935. doi:10.1111/dom.12494.

223. Briand F , Mayoux E , Brousseau E , et al. Empagliflozin, via switching metabolism toward lipid utilization, moderately increases LDL cholesterol levels through reduced LDL catabolism. Diabetes . 2016;65(7):2032-2038. doi:10.2337/db16-0049 27207551.

224. Tang H , Zhang X , Zhang J , et al. Elevated serum magnesium associated with SGLT2 inhibitor use in type 2 diabetes patients: a meta-analysis of randomised controlled trials. Diabetologia . 2016;59(12):2546–2551. doi:10.1007/s00125-016-4101-6 27628105.

225. Forst T , Guthrie R , Goldenberg R , et al. Efficacy and safety of canagliflozin over 52 weeks in patients with type 2 diabetes on background metformin and pioglitazone. Diabetes Obesity Metab . 2014;16(5):467–477. doi:10.1111/dom.12273.

226. Weir MR , Kline I , Xie J , et al. Effect of canagliflozin on serum electrolytes in patients with type 2 diabetes in relation to estimated glomerular filtration rate (eGFR). Curr Med Res Opin . 2014;30(9):1759–1768. doi:10.1185/03007995.2014.919907 24786834.

227. Taylor SI , Blau JE , Rother KI . Possible adverse effects of SGLT2 inhibitors on bone. Lancet Diabetes Endocrinol . 2015;3(1):8-10. doi:10.1016/s2213-8587(14)70227-x 25523498.

228. Armstrong GP. Empagliflozin-Mediated Lithium Excretion: A Case Study and Clinical Applications. Am J Case Rep. 2020 Jun 10;21:e923311.

229. Devineni D, Manitpisitkul P, Vaccaro N, Bernard A, Skee D, Mamidi RN, Tian H, Weiner S, Stieltjes H, Sha S, Rothenberg P. Effect of canagliflozin, a sodium glucose co-transporter 2 inhibitor, on the pharmacokinetics of oral contraceptives, warfarin, and digoxin in healthy participants. Int J Clin Pharmacol Ther. 2015 Jan;53(1):41-53.

230. Scheen AJ. Drug-drug interactions with sodium-glucose cotransporters type 2 (SGLT2) inhibitors, new oral glucose-lowering agents for the management of type 2 diabetes mellitus. Clin Pharmacokinet. 2014 Apr;53(4):295-304.

231. Vallon V. The mechanisms and therapeutic potential of SGLT2 inhibitors in diabetes mellitus. Annu Rev Med. 2015;66:255-70.

232. Kim WJ, Park CY. 1,5-Anhydroglucitol in diabetes mellitus. Endocrine. 2013 Feb;43(1):33-40.

233. Deedwania P. Hypertension, dyslipidemia, and insulin resistance in patients with diabetes mellitus or the cardiometabolic syndrome: benefits of vasodilating β-blockers. J Clin Hypertens (Greenwich). 2011 Jan;13(1):52-9.

234 Schaeffer SE, DesLauriers C, Spiller HA, Aleguas A, Baeza S, Ryan ML. Retrospective review of SGLT2 inhibitor exposures reported to 13 poison centers. Clin Toxicol (Phila). 2018 Mar;56(3):204-208.

235. Baig MA, Nogar J. Euglycemia despite a sodium glucose co-transporter 2 inhibitor overdose. World J Emerg Med. 2022;13(2):147-148.

236. EASL-EASD-EASO Clinical Practice Guidelines for the management of non-alcoholic fatty liver disease. J Hepatol . 2016;64(6):1388–1402. doi:10.1016/j.jhep.2015.11.004 27062661.

237. Saponaro C , Gaggini M , Gastaldelli A . Nonalcoholic fatty liver disease and type 2 diabetes: common pathophysiologic mechanisms. Curr Diab Rep . 2015;15:6. doi:10.1007/s11892-015-0607-4.

238. Younossi ZM , Koenig AB , Abdelatif D , et al. Global epidemiology of nonalcoholic fatty liver disease-meta-analytic assessment of prevalence, incidence, and outcomes. Hepatology . 2016;64:73-84. doi:10.1002/hep.28431 26707365.

239. Seko Y , Sumida Y , Tanaka S , et al. Serum alanine aminotransferase predicts the histological course of non-alcoholic steatohepatitis in Japanese patients. Hepatol Res . 2014;45:10. doi:10.1111/hepr.12456 24606181.

240. Seko Y , Nishikawa T , Umemura A , et al. Efficacy and safety of canagliflozin in type 2 diabetes mellitus patients with biopsy-proven nonalcoholic steatohepatitis classified as stage 1-3 fibrosis. Diabetes Metab Syndrome Obesity . 2018;(2018(11):835-843. doi:10.2147/dmso.s184767.

241. Kabil SL , Mahmoud NM . Canagliflozin protects against non-alcoholic steatohepatitis in type-2 diabetic rats through zinc alpha-2 glycoprotein up-regulation. Eur J Pharmacol . 2018;828:135-145. doi:10.1016/j.ejphar.2018.03.043 29608898.

242. Zaccardi F , Webb DR , Htike ZZ , et al. Efficacy and safety of sodium-glucose co-transporter-2 inhibitors in type 2 diabetes mellitus: systematic review and network meta-analysis. Diabetes Obesity Metab . 2016;18(8):783–794. doi:10.1111/dom.12670.

243. Ferrannini G , Hach T , Crowe S , Sanghvi A , Hall KD , Ferrannini E . Energy balance after sodium-glucose cotransporter 2 inhibition. Diabetes Care . 2015;38(9):1730-1735. doi:10.2337/dc15-0355 26180105.

244. He YL , Haynes W , Meyers CD , et al. The effects of licogliflozin, a dual SGLT1/2 inhibitor, on body weight in obese patients with or without diabetes. Diabetes Obesity Metab . 2019. doi:10.1111/dom.13654.

245. Scafoglio CR , Villegas B , Abdelhady G , et al. Sodium-glucose transporter 2 is a diagnostic and therapeutic target for early-stage lung adenocarcinoma. Sci Transl Med . 2018;10:467. doi:10.1126/scitranslmed.aat5933.

246. Park SW , Goodpaster BH , Lee JS , et al. Excessive loss of skeletal muscle mass in older adults with type 2 diabetes. Diabetes Care . 2009;32(11):1993-1997. doi:10.2337/dc09-0264 19549734.

247. Özdirenç M , Biberoğlu S , Özcan A . Evaluation of physical fitness in patients with Type 2 diabetes mellitus. Diabetes Res Clin Pract . 2003;60(3):171–176. doi:10.1016/s0168-8227(03)00064-0 12757989.

248. Regensteiner JG , Bauer TA , Reusch JE . Rosiglitazone improves exercise capacity in individuals with type 2 diabetes. Diabetes Care . 2005;28(12):2877–2883. doi:10.2337/diacare.28.12.2877 16306548.

249. Kadoglou NPE , Iliadis F , Angelopoulou N , et al. Beneficial effects of rosiglitazone on novel cardiovascular risk factors in patients with type 2 diabetes mellitus. Diabetic Med . 2008;25(3):333-340. doi:10.1111/j.1464-5491.2007.02375.x 18307460.

250. Lepore JJ , Olson E , Demopoulos L , et al. Effects of the novel long-acting GLP-1 agonist, albiglutide, on cardiac function, cardiac metabolism, and exercise capacity in patients with chronic heart failure and reduced ejection fraction. JACC . 2016;4(7):559-566. doi:10.1016/j.jchf.2016.01.008 27039125.

251. Núñez J , Palau P , Domínguez E , et al. Early effects of empagliflozin on exercise tolerance in patients with heart failure: a pilot study. Clin Cardiol . 2018;41(4):476-480. doi:10.1002/clc.22899 29663436.

252. Carbone S , Canada JM , Billingsley HE , et al. Effects of empagliflozin on cardiorespiratory fitness and significant interaction of loop diuretics. Diabetes Obesity Metab . 2018;20(8):2014–2018. doi:10.1111/dom.13309.

253. Washburn WN , Poucher SM . Differentiating sodium-glucose co-transporter-2 inhibitors in development for the treatment of type 2 diabetes mellitus. Expert Opin Investig Drugs . 2013;22(4):463–486. doi:10.1517/13543784.2013.774372.

254. Cefalo CMA , Cinti F , Moffa S , et al. Sotagliflozin, the first dual SGLT inhibitor: current outlook and perspectives. Cardiovasc Diabetol . 2019;18:1. doi:10.1186/s12933-019-0828-y 30626440.

255. Rieg JAD , Rieg T . What does sodium-glucose co-transporter 1 inhibition add: prospects for dual inhibition. Diabetes Obesity Metab . 2019;21(S2):43–52. doi:10.1111/dom.13630.

256. Zambrowicz B , Freiman J , Brown PM , et al. LX4211, a dual SGLT1/SGLT2 inhibitor, improved glycemic control in patients with type 2 diabetes in a randomized, placebo-controlled trial. Clin Pharmacol Ther . 2012;92(2):158-169. doi:10.1038/clpt.2012.58 22739142.

257. Zambrowicz B , Lapuerta P , Strumph P , et al. LX4211 therapy reduces postprandial glucose levels in patients with type 2 diabetes mellitus and renal impairment despite low urinary glucose excretion. Clin Ther . 2015;37:1. doi:10.1016/j.clinthera.2014.10.026 25592086.

258. Garg SK , Henry RR , Banks P , et al. Effects of sotagliflozin added to insulin in patients with type 1 diabetes. N Engl J Med . 2017;377(24):2337-2348. doi:10.1056/nejmoa1708337 28899222.

SUMMARY

Sodium-glucose cotransporter 2 (SGLT2) inhibitors, initially developed as a new class of anti-hyperglycemic drugs, have been shown to significantly improve metabolic indicators and protect the kidneys and heart of patients with and without type 2 diabetes. The possible mechanisms of these unexpected cardio-renal benefits are the subject of extensive research, as they cannot be attributed solely to improved glycemic control. In particular, emerging data indicate that metabolic reprogramming is involved in the progression of cardio-renal metabolic diseases. SGLT2 inhibitors reprogram systemic metabolism towards a fasting-type metabolic paradigm, involving the metabolic switch from carbohydrates to other energy substrates and the regulation of associated nutrient elimination pathways, which may explain some of their protective effects on the cardio-adrenal system. In this book, we will focus on the current understanding of cardio-renal protection by SGLT2 inhibitors, explaining the pathophysiological mechanisms involved, and outline the largest trials that have demonstrated this organoprotective effect.

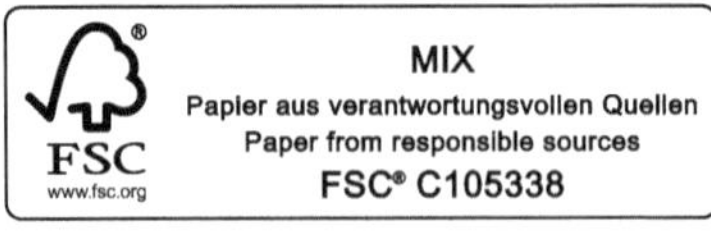

Printed by Books on Demand GmbH, Norderstedt / Germany